**2024 EDITION**

**+4 Weeks MEAL PLAN**

# RHEUMATOID ARTHRITIS DIET

## COOKBOOK FOR WOMEN

### Wholesome Recipes to Manage Inflammatory Flare-Ups and Fatigue

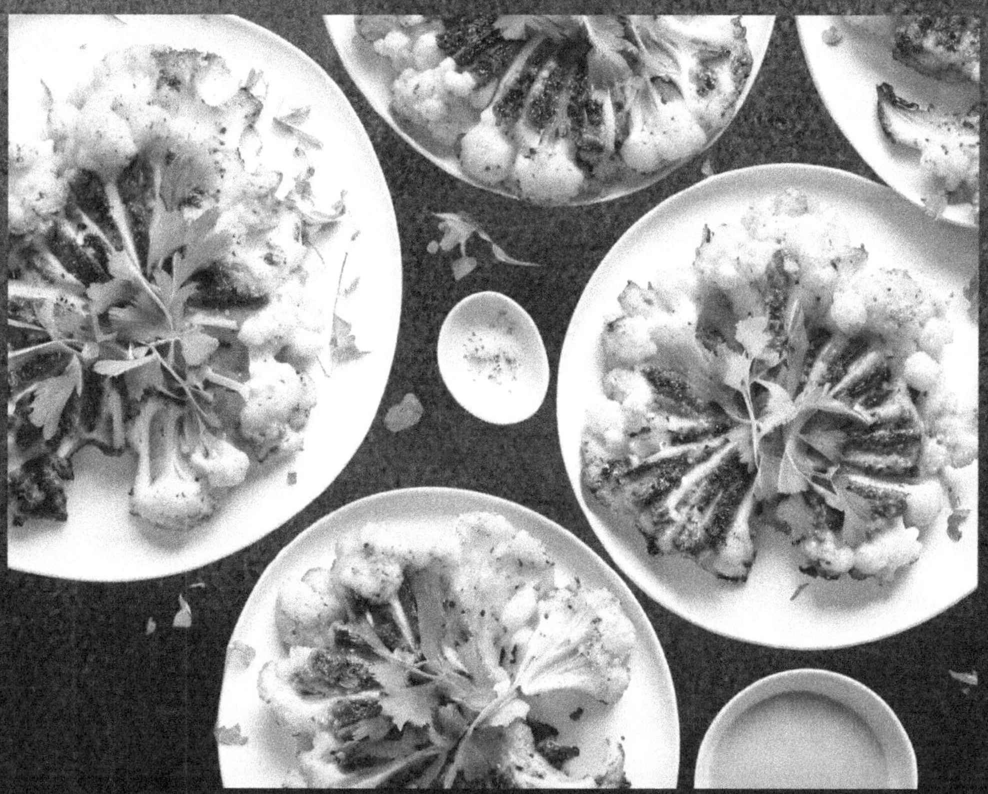

**Judy Kelly**

# Table of Contents

# Introduction

Welcome to "A Rheumatoid Arthritis Cookbook for Women"! This cookbook is designed to empower women living with rheumatoid arthritis to take control of their health through nourishing and delicious recipes. Rheumatoid arthritis is a chronic autoimmune condition that primarily affects the joints, and women are more likely than men to develop this condition.

Living with rheumatoid arthritis can be challenging, as the symptoms such as joint pain, inflammation, and fatigue can impact daily life. However, research suggests that diet can play a significant role in managing the symptoms of rheumatoid arthritis and improving overall well-being.

In this cookbook, you'll find a variety of recipes that are not only flavorful and satisfying but also packed with nutrients that can help reduce inflammation and boost energy levels. From hearty breakfasts to comforting dinners and indulgent desserts, each recipe is thoughtfully crafted to support women with rheumatoid arthritis.

But this cookbook is more than just a collection of recipes. It's a guide to help you make informed choices about the foods you eat and how they can impact your health. You'll find tips on meal planning, ingredient selection, and how to incorporate these recipes into your daily life.

Whether you're looking for simple and nutritious meals or elegant dishes for special occasions, this cookbook is here to inspire and support you on your journey to better health. So, let's get cooking and discover how delicious and nutritious meals can help you manage rheumatoid arthritis and thrive as a woman.

## - About Rheumatoid Arthritis and Women's Health

Rheumatoid arthritis (RA) is an autoimmune disease that causes chronic inflammation of the joints. It can lead to pain, swelling, stiffness, and loss of function in the affected joints. While RA can affect people of all ages and genders, it is more common in women, with women being two to three times more likely to develop RA than men.

The reasons for this gender difference are not entirely clear, but researchers believe that hormones, genetics, and environmental factors may all play a role. For example, some studies suggest that the female hormone estrogen may influence the immune system and contribute to the development of RA.

Women with RA may also face unique challenges related to their health. For example, RA can affect women's reproductive health, including their ability to conceive and carry a pregnancy to term. Additionally, women with RA may be at increased risk for certain other health conditions, such as osteoporosis and heart disease.

Managing RA requires a comprehensive approach that may include medication, physical therapy, and lifestyle changes. Diet can also play a crucial role in managing the symptoms of RA and supporting overall health. By making smart food choices, women with RA can help reduce inflammation, boost their energy levels, and improve their quality of life.

## - How Diet Can Help Manage Symptoms

Diet plays a crucial role in managing the symptoms of rheumatoid arthritis (RA) and supporting overall health. While diet alone cannot cure RA, it can help reduce inflammation, boost energy levels, and improve overall well-being. Here are some ways in which diet can help manage the symptoms of RA:

1. Anti-inflammatory foods: Incorporating anti-inflammatory foods into your diet can help reduce inflammation in the body. These include foods rich in omega-3 fatty acids (such as fatty fish like salmon and sardines, flaxseeds, and walnuts), fruits and vegetables (especially berries, cherries, and leafy greens), and spices (such as turmeric and ginger).

2. Healthy fats: Including healthy fats in your diet, such as those found in olive oil, avocados, and nuts, can help reduce inflammation and improve joint health.

3. Protein: Getting an adequate amount of protein is important for maintaining muscle mass and strength, which can help support joint health. Good sources of protein include lean meats, poultry, fish, eggs, dairy products, legumes, and tofu.

4. Whole grains: Whole grains like brown rice, quinoa, oats, and whole wheat provide fiber and important nutrients that can help support overall health and reduce inflammation.

5. Limiting processed foods and sugar: Processed foods and foods high in sugar can contribute to inflammation in the body. Limiting these foods can help manage symptoms of RA.

6. Hydration: Staying hydrated is important for overall health and can help reduce joint pain and stiffness.

It's important to note that while diet can play a significant role in managing RA, it is not a substitute for medical treatment. It's always best to work with a healthcare provider or dietitian to develop a diet plan that is tailored to your individual needs and health goals.

# Chapter 1: Energizing Breakfasts

1. Anti-Inflammatory Smoothie Bowl
   - Ingredients:
     - 1/2 cup frozen mixed berries
     - 1/2 banana
     - 1/2 cup spinach
     - 1/2 cup almond milk
     - 1 tbsp chia seeds
     - 1 tbsp almond butter
     - Toppings: sliced almonds, shredded coconut, fresh berries

   - Instructions:
     1. Blend berries, banana, spinach, almond milk, chia seeds, and almond butter until smooth.
     2. Pour into a bowl and top with sliced almonds, shredded coconut, and fresh berries.

2. Turmeric Porridge with Berries
   - Ingredients:
     - 1/2 cup rolled oats
     - 1 cup almond milk
     - 1/2 tsp turmeric powder
     - 1/2 tsp cinnamon
     - 1/2 tsp vanilla extract
     - Toppings: mixed berries, honey, chopped nuts

   - Instructions:
     1. In a saucepan, combine oats, almond milk, turmeric, cinnamon, and vanilla.
     2. Cook over medium heat, stirring occasionally, until thickened.
     3. Serve topped with mixed berries, honey, and chopped nuts.

3. Avocado Toast with Chickpea Mash
   - Ingredients:
     - 1 ripe avocado
     - 1/2 lemon, juiced
     - 1/2 can chickpeas, drained and rinsed
     - 1 tbsp tahini
     - 1/2 tsp cumin
     - 2 slices whole grain bread, toasted

   - Instructions:
     1. In a bowl, mash avocado with lemon juice and a pinch of salt.
     2. In another bowl, mash chickpeas with tahini, cumin, and a splash of water.
     3. Spread avocado mixture on toast, top with chickpea mash, and sprinkle with additional cumin if desired.

4. Chia Seed Pudding with Mixed Berries
   - Ingredients:
     - 2 tbsp chia seeds
     - 1/2 cup almond milk
     - 1/2 tsp vanilla extract
     - 1 tbsp honey
     - 1/2 cup mixed berries

   - Instructions:
     1. In a bowl, combine chia seeds, almond milk, vanilla, and honey. Stir well.
     2. Cover and refrigerate overnight.
     3. In the morning, top with mixed berries before serving.

5. Oatmeal with Almond Butter and Banana
   - Ingredients:
     - 1/2 cup rolled oats

- 1 cup almond milk
- 1/2 banana, sliced
- 1 tbsp almond butter
- 1 tbsp honey
- 1/2 tsp cinnamon

- Instructions:
    1. In a saucepan, combine oats and almond milk. Cook over medium heat until thickened.
    2. Stir in banana, almond butter, honey, and cinnamon.
    3. Cook for another minute, then serve hot.

6. Greek Yogurt Parfait with Granola and Berries
   - Ingredients:
     - 1/2 cup Greek yogurt
     - 1/4 cup granola
     - 1/4 cup mixed berries
     - 1 tbsp honey

   - Instructions:
     1. In a glass, layer Greek yogurt, granola, and mixed berries.
     2. Drizzle with honey before serving.

7. Egg and Veggie Scramble
   - Ingredients:
     - 2 eggs
     - 1/2 cup mixed veggies (bell peppers, onions, spinach)
     - 1/2 tbsp olive oil
     - Salt and pepper to taste

   - Instructions:
     1. In a pan, heat olive oil over medium heat. Add veggies and sauté until tender.

2. In a bowl, whisk eggs with salt and pepper. Pour over veggies and scramble until cooked through.


8. Sweet Potato Breakfast Hash
   - Ingredients:
     - 1 sweet potato, diced
     - 1/2 onion, diced
     - 1/2 bell pepper, diced
     - 1/2 tbsp olive oil
     - 1/2 tsp paprika
     - 1/2 tsp cumin
     - Salt and pepper to taste

   - Instructions:
     1. In a pan, heat olive oil over medium heat. Add sweet potato, onion, and bell pepper.
     2. Season with paprika, cumin, salt, and pepper. Cook until sweet potato is tender and slightly crispy.


9. Banana Nut Overnight Oats
   - Ingredients:
     - 1/2 cup rolled oats
     - 1/2 cup almond milk
     - 1/2 banana, mashed
     - 1 tbsp chopped nuts
     - 1/2 tbsp honey
     - 1/2 tsp cinnamon

   - Instructions:
     1. In a jar, combine oats, almond milk, banana, nuts, honey, and cinnamon. Stir well.
     2. Cover and refrigerate overnight. Stir before serving.

10. Berry and Spinach Smoothie
   - Ingredients:
     - 1/2 cup mixed berries
     - 1/2 banana
     - 1/2 cup spinach
     - 1/2 cup almond milk
     - 1 tbsp chia seeds

   - Instructions:
     1. Blend berries, banana, spinach, almond milk, and chia seeds until smooth.
     2. Pour into a glass and serve cold.

11. Coconut Chia Seed Pudding
   - Ingredients:
     - 2 tbsp chia seeds
     - 1/2 cup coconut milk
     - 1/2 tsp vanilla extract
     - 1/2 tbsp honey
     - Shredded coconut for topping

   - Instructions:
     1. In a bowl, combine chia seeds, coconut milk, vanilla, and honey. Stir well.
     2. Cover and refrigerate for at least 1 hour or overnight.
     3. Top with shredded coconut before serving.

12. Apple Cinnamon Baked Oatmeal
   - Ingredients:
     - 1/2 cup rolled oats
     - 1/2 cup almond milk
     - 1/2 apple, diced
     - 1/2 tbsp honey

- 1/2 tsp cinnamon

- Instructions:
   1. Preheat oven to 350°F (175°C).
   2. In a bowl, combine oats, almond milk, apple, honey, and cinnamon. Stir well.
   3. Pour mixture into a greased baking dish and bake for 25-30 minutes, or until set.

13. Spinach and Mushroom Omelette
   - Ingredients:
     - 2 eggs
     - 1/2 cup spinach, chopped
     - 1/4 cup mushrooms, sliced
     - 1/4 cup shredded cheese
     - Salt and pepper to taste

   - Instructions:
   1. In a bowl, whisk eggs with salt and pepper.
   2. In a pan, sauté spinach and mushrooms until tender. Pour eggs over veggies and cook until set.
   3. Sprinkle with cheese and fold over before serving.

14. Quinoa Breakfast Bowl
   - Ingredients:
     - 1/2 cup cooked quinoa
     - 1/2 cup almond milk
     - 1/2 banana, sliced
     - 1 tbsp almond butter
     - 1 tbsp honey
     - 1/2 tsp cinnamon

   - Instructions:

    1. In a bowl, combine quinoa, almond milk, banana, almond butter, honey, and cinnamon. Stir well.

    2. Microwave for 1-2 minutes, or until heated through. Stir before serving.

15. Greek Yogurt Pancakes
   - Ingredients:
     - 1/2 cup Greek yogurt
     - 1 egg
     - 1/4 cup almond milk
     - 1/2 cup whole wheat flour
     - 1/2 tsp baking powder
     - 1/2 tsp cinnamon

   - Instructions:
     1. In a bowl, whisk together Greek yogurt, egg, and almond milk.
     2. Add flour, baking powder, and cinnamon. Stir until smooth.
     3. Heat a pan over medium heat and pour batter to form pancakes. Cook until bubbles form, then flip and cook until golden brown.

16. Blueberry Almond Baked Oatmeal Cups
   - Ingredients:
     - 1 cup rolled oats
     - 1/2 cup almond milk
     - 1/2 cup blueberries
     - 1/4 cup chopped almonds
     - 1/2 tbsp honey
     - 1/2 tsp vanilla extract

   - Instructions:
     1. Preheat oven to 350°F (175°C) and grease a muffin tin.
     2. In a bowl, combine oats, almond milk, blueberries, almonds, honey, and vanilla. Stir well.

3. Divide mixture into muffin cups and bake for 20-25 minutes, or until set.

17. Peanut Butter Banana Overnight Oats
   - Ingredients:
     - 1/2 cup rolled oats
     - 1/2 cup almond milk
     - 1/2 banana, mashed
     - 1 tbsp peanut butter
     - 1/2 tbsp honey
     - 1/2 tsp vanilla extract

   - Instructions:
     1. In a jar, combine oats, almond milk, banana, peanut butter, honey, and vanilla. Stir well.
     2. Cover and refrigerate overnight. Stir before serving.

18. Almond Flour Banana Muffins
   - Ingredients:
     - 1 1/2 cups almond flour
     - 1/2 tsp baking powder
     - 1/2 tsp baking soda
     - 1/2 tsp cinnamon
     - 2 ripe bananas, mashed
     - 2 eggs
     - 1/4 cup almond milk
     - 1/4 cup honey

   - Instructions:
     1. Preheat oven to 350°F (175°C) and line a muffin tin with liners.
     2. In a bowl, combine almond flour, baking powder, baking soda, and cinnamon.

3. In another bowl, whisk together bananas, eggs, almond milk, and honey.

4. Add wet ingredients to dry ingredients and stir until combined. Divide batter into muffin cups and bake for 20-25 minutes, or until a toothpick inserted into the center comes out clean.

19. Green Smoothie with Avocado
   - Ingredients:
     - 1/2 avocado
     - 1/2 banana
     - 1/2 cup spinach
     - 1/2 cup almond milk
     - 1 tbsp chia seeds
     - 1 tbsp honey

   - Instructions:
     1. Blend avocado, banana, spinach, almond milk, chia seeds, and honey until smooth.
     2. Pour into a glass and serve cold.

20. Veggie Breakfast Burrito
   - Ingredients:
     - 1 whole wheat tortilla
     - 2 eggs, scrambled
     - 1/4 cup black beans, drained and rinsed
     - 1/4 cup diced bell peppers
     - 2 tbsp shredded cheese
     - Salsa and avocado for topping

   - Instructions:
     1. Heat tortilla in a pan over medium heat. Fill with scrambled eggs, black beans, bell peppers, and cheese.
     2. Roll up the tortilla and cook until golden brown on all sides.

3. Top with salsa and avocado before serving.

# Chapter 2: Nourishing Soups and Salads

1. Immune-Boosting Vegetable Soup
   - Ingredients:
     - 1 tbsp olive oil
     - 1 onion, chopped
     - 2 carrots, chopped
     - 2 celery stalks, chopped
     - 2 garlic cloves, minced
     - 1 tsp turmeric
     - 1 tsp cumin
     - 6 cups vegetable broth
     - 1 can (14 oz) diced tomatoes
     - 1 can (14 oz) chickpeas, drained and rinsed
     - 2 cups chopped kale
     - Salt and pepper to taste

   - Instructions:
     1. In a large pot, heat olive oil over medium heat. Add onion, carrots, and celery. Cook until softened, about 5 minutes.
     2. Add garlic, turmeric, and cumin. Cook for another minute.
     3. Add vegetable broth, diced tomatoes, and chickpeas. Bring to a simmer and cook for 15 minutes.
     4. Stir in kale and cook until wilted, about 5 minutes. Season with salt and pepper.

2. Quinoa Salad with Roasted Vegetables
   - Ingredients:
     - 1 cup quinoa
     - 2 cups water
     - 1 red bell pepper, chopped
     - 1 zucchini, chopped
     - 1 yellow squash, chopped

- 1 red onion, sliced
- 2 tbsp olive oil
- 1 tsp dried thyme
- Salt and pepper to taste
- 1/4 cup chopped fresh parsley
- 1/4 cup lemon juice
- 1/4 cup olive oil

- Instructions:
1. Preheat oven to 400°F (200°C).
2. In a large bowl, toss bell pepper, zucchini, squash, and onion with olive oil, thyme, salt, and pepper. Spread on a baking sheet.
3. Roast vegetables in the preheated oven for 25-30 minutes, or until tender and slightly caramelized. Let cool.
4. In a medium saucepan, combine quinoa and water. Bring to a boil, then reduce heat and simmer for 15 minutes, or until quinoa is tender and water is absorbed.
5. In a large bowl, combine cooked quinoa, roasted vegetables, parsley, lemon juice, and olive oil. Toss to combine. Season with additional salt and pepper if needed.

3. Spinach and Strawberry Salad with Walnuts
  - Ingredients:
    - 4 cups baby spinach
    - 1 cup sliced strawberries
    - 1/4 cup chopped walnuts
    - 2 tbsp balsamic vinegar
    - 1 tbsp olive oil
    - 1 tsp honey
    - Salt and pepper to taste

  - Instructions:
1. In a large bowl, combine baby spinach, strawberries, and walnuts.

2. In a small bowl, whisk together balsamic vinegar, olive oil, honey, salt, and pepper.

3. Drizzle dressing over salad and toss to combine.


4. Coconut Curry Lentil Soup
  - Ingredients:
    - 1 tbsp coconut oil
    - 1 onion, chopped
    - 2 carrots, chopped
    - 2 celery stalks, chopped
    - 3 garlic cloves, minced
    - 1 tbsp curry powder
    - 1 tsp turmeric
    - 1 cup red lentils
    - 4 cups vegetable broth
    - 1 can (14 oz) coconut milk
    - Salt and pepper to taste
    - Fresh cilantro for garnish

  - Instructions:
    1. In a large pot, heat coconut oil over medium heat. Add onion, carrots, and celery. Cook until softened, about 5 minutes.

2. Add garlic, curry powder, and turmeric. Cook for another minute.

3. Add lentils and vegetable broth. Bring to a simmer and cook for 20-25 minutes, or until lentils are tender.

4. Stir in coconut milk and heat through. Season with salt and pepper. Garnish with fresh cilantro before serving.


5. Roasted Butternut Squash Soup
  - Ingredients:
    - 1 butternut squash, peeled, seeded, and cubed
    - 1 onion, chopped
    - 2 carrots, chopped

- 2 celery stalks, chopped
- 3 garlic cloves, minced
- 2 tbsp olive oil
- 4 cups vegetable broth
- 1 tsp dried thyme
- Salt and pepper to taste
- Coconut cream for garnish

- Instructions:
1. Preheat oven to 400°F (200°C).
2. In a large bowl, toss butternut squash, onion, carrots, celery, and garlic with olive oil. Spread on a baking sheet.
3. Roast vegetables in the preheated oven for 30-40 minutes, or until tender and slightly caramelized.
4. In a large pot, combine roasted vegetables, vegetable broth, thyme, salt, and pepper. Bring to a simmer and cook for 10-15 minutes.
5. Use an immersion blender to blend soup until smooth. Alternatively, blend in batches in a regular blender.
6. Serve hot, garnished with a swirl of coconut cream.

6. Chickpea and Spinach Salad
   - Ingredients:
   - 1 can (14 oz) chickpeas, drained and rinsed
   - 4 cups baby spinach
   - 1/2 red onion, thinly sliced
   - 1/4 cup crumbled feta cheese
   - 2 tbsp olive oil
   - 1 tbsp lemon juice
   - 1 tsp Dijon mustard
   - Salt and pepper to taste

   - Instructions:

1. In a large bowl, combine chickpeas, spinach, red onion, and feta cheese.

2. In a small bowl, whisk together olive oil, lemon juice, Dijon mustard, salt, and pepper.

3. Drizzle dressing over salad and toss to combine.

7. Kale and Quinoa Salad
   - Ingredients:
     - 1 cup cooked quinoa
     - 4 cups chopped kale
     - 1/4 cup dried cranberries
     - 1/4 cup chopped walnuts
     - 2 tbsp olive oil
     - 1 tbsp balsamic vinegar
     - 1 tsp honey
     - Salt and pepper to taste

   - Instructions:
     1. In a large bowl, combine quinoa, kale, cranberries, and walnuts.
     2. In a small bowl, whisk together olive oil, balsamic vinegar, honey, salt, and pepper.
     3. Drizzle dressing over salad and toss to combine.

8. Miso Soup with Tofu and Vegetables
   - Ingredients:
     - 4 cups vegetable broth
     - 2 tbsp miso paste
     - 1 cup cubed tofu
     - 1 cup sliced mushrooms
     - 1/2 cup sliced green onions
     - 1/2 cup shredded cabbage
     - 1 tbsp soy sauce
     - 1 tsp sesame oil

- Instructions:
    1. In a large pot, bring vegetable broth to a simmer.
    2. In a small bowl, whisk together miso paste and a small amount of hot broth until smooth. Stir miso mixture into the pot.
    3. Add tofu, mushrooms, green onions, and cabbage. Cook for 5-7 minutes, or until vegetables are tender.
    4. Stir in soy sauce and sesame oil. Serve hot.

9. Greek Chickpea Salad
  - Ingredients:
    - 1 can (14 oz) chickpeas, drained and rinsed
    - 1 cucumber, diced
    - 1 bell pepper, diced
    - 1/4 cup chopped red onion
    - 1/4 cup chopped fresh parsley
    - 1/4 cup crumbled feta cheese
    - 2 tbsp olive oil
    - 1 tbsp lemon juice
    - 1 tsp dried oregano
    - Salt and pepper to taste

  - Instructions:
    1. In a large bowl, combine chickpeas, cucumber, bell pepper, red onion, parsley, and feta cheese.
    2. In a small bowl, whisk together olive oil, lemon juice, oregano, salt, and pepper.
    3. Drizzle dressing over salad and toss to combine.

10. Tomato Basil Soup
  - Ingredients:
    - 1 tbsp olive oil
    - 1 onion, chopped

- 2 carrots, chopped
- 2 celery stalks, chopped
- 3 garlic cloves, minced
- 1 can (28 oz) diced tomatoes
- 4 cups vegetable broth
- 1/4 cup chopped fresh basil
- Salt and pepper to taste
- Coconut cream for garnish

- Instructions:
  1. In a large pot, heat olive oil over medium heat. Add onion, carrots, and celery. Cook until softened, about 5 minutes.
  2. Add garlic and cook for another minute.
  3. Add diced tomatoes (with juices) and vegetable broth. Bring to a simmer and cook for 15-20 minutes.
  4. Stir in fresh basil. Use an immersion blender to blend soup until smooth. Alternatively, blend in batches in a regular blender.
  5. Season with salt and pepper. Serve hot, garnished with a swirl of coconut cream.

11. Cabbage and White Bean Soup
  - Ingredients:
    - 1 tbsp olive oil
    - 1 onion, chopped
    - 2 carrots, chopped
    - 2 celery stalks, chopped
    - 3 garlic cloves, minced
    - 1 small cabbage, shredded
    - 1 can (14 oz) white beans, drained and rinsed
    - 4 cups vegetable broth
    - 1 tsp dried thyme
    - Salt and pepper to taste
    - Fresh parsley for garnish

- Instructions:
    1. In a large pot, heat olive oil over medium heat. Add onion, carrots, celery, and garlic. Cook until softened, about 5 minutes.
    2. Add cabbage and cook for another 5 minutes.
    3. Add white beans, vegetable broth, thyme, salt, and pepper. Bring to a simmer and cook for 15-20 minutes.
    4. Serve hot, garnished with fresh parsley.

12. Asian-Inspired Broccoli Salad
   - Ingredients:
     - 4 cups chopped broccoli
     - 1/4 cup sliced almonds
     - 1/4 cup dried cranberries
     - 2 green onions, sliced
     - 2 tbsp soy sauce
     - 1 tbsp rice vinegar
     - 1 tbsp sesame oil
     - 1 tsp honey
     - 1/2 tsp grated ginger

   - Instructions:
     1. In a large bowl, combine broccoli, almonds, cranberries, and green onions.
     2. In a small bowl, whisk together soy sauce, rice vinegar, sesame oil, honey, and ginger.
     3. Drizzle dressing over salad and toss to combine.

13. Mediterranean Chickpea Salad
   - Ingredients:
     - 1 can (14 oz) chickpeas, drained and rinsed
     - 1 cucumber, diced
     - 1 bell pepper, diced

- 1/4 cup chopped red onion
- 1/4 cup chopped fresh parsley
- 1/4 cup crumbled feta cheese
- 2 tbsp olive oil
- 1 tbsp lemon juice
- 1 tsp dried oregano
- Salt and pepper to taste

- Instructions:
  1. In a large bowl, combine chickpeas, cucumber, bell pepper, red onion, parsley, and feta cheese.
  2. In a small bowl, whisk together olive oil, lemon juice, oregano, salt, and pepper.
  3. Drizzle dressing over salad and toss to combine.

14. Lentil and Vegetable Soup
  - Ingredients:
    - 1 tbsp olive oil
    - 1 onion, chopped
    - 2 carrots, chopped
    - 2 celery stalks, chopped
    - 3 garlic cloves, minced
    - 1 tsp ground cumin
    - 1 tsp ground coriander
    - 1 cup dried green lentils, rinsed
    - 4 cups vegetable broth
    - 1 can (14 oz) diced tomatoes
    - 2 cups chopped spinach
    - Salt and pepper to taste

  - Instructions:
    1. In a large pot, heat olive oil over medium heat. Add onion, carrots, celery, and garlic. Cook until softened, about 5 minutes.

2. Add cumin and coriander. Cook for another minute.

3. Add lentils, vegetable broth, and diced tomatoes. Bring to a simmer and cook for 20-25 minutes, or until lentils are tender.

4. Stir in spinach and cook until wilted. Season with salt and pepper.

15. Roasted Vegetable Salad
   - Ingredients:
      - 2 cups chopped mixed vegetables (bell peppers, zucchini, eggplant, cherry tomatoes)
      - 1 tbsp olive oil
      - 1 tsp dried herbs (such as thyme or rosemary)
      - Salt and pepper to taste
      - 4 cups mixed greens
      - 1/4 cup crumbled goat cheese
      - Balsamic glaze for drizzling

   - Instructions:
      1. Preheat oven to 400°F (200°C).
      2. In a large bowl, toss mixed vegetables with olive oil, dried herbs, salt, and pepper. Spread on a baking sheet.
      3. Roast vegetables in the preheated oven for 20-25 minutes, or until tender and slightly caramelized. Let cool.
      4. In a large bowl, combine mixed greens and roasted vegetables. Top with crumbled goat cheese and drizzle with balsamic glaze.

16. Spiced Carrot Soup
   - Ingredients:
      - 1 tbsp olive oil
      - 1 onion, chopped
      - 2 garlic cloves, minced
      - 1 tsp ground cumin
      - 1/2 tsp ground coriander

- 1/4 tsp ground cinnamon
- 1 lb carrots, peeled and chopped
- 4 cups vegetable broth
- 1/2 cup coconut milk
- Salt and pepper to taste
- Fresh cilantro for garnish

- Instructions:
1. In a large pot, heat olive oil over medium heat. Add onion and garlic. Cook until softened, about 5 minutes.
2. Add cumin, coriander, and cinnamon. Cook for another minute.
3. Add carrots and vegetable broth. Bring to a simmer and cook for 20-25 minutes, or until carrots are tender.
4. Use an immersion blender to blend soup until smooth. Alternatively, blend in batches in a regular blender.
5. Stir in coconut milk. Season with salt and pepper. Serve hot, garnished with fresh cilantro.

17. Greek Orzo Salad
  - Ingredients:
    - 1 cup orzo, cooked and cooled
    - 1 cucumber, diced
    - 1 bell pepper, diced
    - 1/4 cup sliced black olives
    - 1/4 cup crumbled feta cheese
    - 2 tbsp chopped fresh parsley
    - 2 tbsp olive oil
    - 1 tbsp lemon juice
    - 1 tsp dried oregano
    - Salt and pepper to taste

  - Instructions:

1. In a large bowl, combine cooked orzo, cucumber, bell pepper, black olives, feta cheese, and parsley.

2. In a small bowl, whisk together olive oil, lemon juice, oregano, salt, and pepper.

3. Drizzle dressing over salad and toss to combine.

18. Creamy Cauliflower Soup
  - Ingredients:
    - 1 tbsp olive oil
    - 1 onion, chopped
    - 2 garlic cloves, minced
    - 1 head cauliflower, chopped
    - 4 cups vegetable broth
    - 1/2 cup coconut milk
    - Salt and pepper to taste
    - Fresh chives for garnish

  - Instructions:
    1. In a large pot, heat olive oil over medium heat. Add onion and garlic. Cook until softened, about 5 minutes.

    2. Add cauliflower and vegetable broth. Bring to a simmer and cook for 20-25 minutes, or until cauliflower is tender.

    3. Use an immersion blender to blend soup until smooth. Alternatively, blend in batches in a regular blender.

    4. Stir in coconut milk. Season with salt and pepper. Serve hot, garnished with fresh chives.

19. Apple Walnut Salad with Maple Dijon Dressing
  - Ingredients:
    - 4 cups mixed greens
    - 1 apple, thinly sliced
    - 1/4 cup chopped walnuts
    - 2 tbsp dried cranberries

- 2 tbsp olive oil
- 1 tbsp apple cider vinegar
- 1 tbsp maple syrup
- 1 tsp Dijon mustard
- Salt and pepper to taste

- Instructions:
  1. In a large bowl, combine mixed greens, apple slices, walnuts, and dried cranberries.
  2. In a small bowl, whisk together olive oil, apple cider vinegar, maple syrup, Dijon mustard, salt, and pepper.
  3. Drizzle dressing over salad and toss to combine.

20. Spicy Black Bean Soup
  - Ingredients:
    - 1 tbsp olive oil
    - 1 onion, chopped
    - 2 garlic cloves, minced
    - 1 red bell pepper, chopped
    - 1 jalapeño pepper, seeded and chopped
    - 1 tbsp chili powder
    - 1 tsp ground cumin
    - 1 can (14 oz) black beans, drained and rinsed
    - 4 cups vegetable broth
    - 1 can (14 oz) diced tomatoes
    - Salt and pepper to taste
    - Fresh cilantro for garnish

  - Instructions:
    1. In a large pot, heat olive oil over medium heat. Add onion, garlic, red bell pepper, and jalapeño pepper. Cook until softened, about 5 minutes.
    2. Add chili powder and cumin. Cook for another minute.

3. Add black beans, vegetable broth, and diced tomatoes. Bring to a simmer and cook for 15-20 minutes.

4. Use an immersion blender to blend soup until partially smooth, leaving some chunks of beans and vegetables. Alternatively, blend in batches in a regular blender.

5. Season with salt and pepper. Serve hot, garnished with fresh cilantro.

# Chapter 3: Wholesome Mains

1. Stuffed Bell Peppers
   - Ingredients:
     - 4 bell peppers
     - 1 tbsp olive oil
     - 1 onion, chopped
     - 2 garlic cloves, minced
     - 1 lb ground turkey
     - 1 can (14 oz) diced tomatoes
     - 1 cup cooked quinoa
     - 1 tsp dried oregano
     - Salt and pepper to taste
     - 1/2 cup shredded cheese

   - Instructions:
     1. Preheat oven to 350°F (175°C).
     2. Cut the tops off the bell peppers and remove the seeds and membranes. Place the peppers in a baking dish.
     3. In a large skillet, heat olive oil over medium heat. Add onion and garlic. Cook until softened, about 5 minutes.
     4. Add ground turkey and cook until browned. Stir in diced tomatoes, quinoa, oregano, salt, and pepper.
     5. Spoon the turkey mixture into the bell peppers. Cover with foil and bake for 30 minutes.
     6. Remove foil, sprinkle with shredded cheese, and bake for an additional 10 minutes, or until cheese is melted and bubbly.

2. Lemon Herb Baked Salmon
   - Ingredients:
     - 4 salmon fillets
     - 2 tbsp olive oil
     - 2 tbsp lemon juice

- 1 tsp dried thyme
- 1 tsp dried rosemary
- 1 tsp dried dill
- Salt and pepper to taste
- Lemon slices for garnish

- Instructions:
1. Preheat oven to 400°F (200°C). Line a baking sheet with parchment paper.
2. Place salmon fillets on the prepared baking sheet.
3. In a small bowl, whisk together olive oil, lemon juice, thyme, rosemary, dill, salt, and pepper.
4. Brush the herb mixture over the salmon fillets.
5. Bake for 12-15 minutes, or until salmon is cooked through and flakes easily with a fork.
6. Serve hot, garnished with lemon slices.

3. Mushroom and Spinach Stuffed Chicken Breast
  - Ingredients:
    - 4 chicken breasts
    - Salt and pepper to taste
    - 1 tbsp olive oil
    - 1 onion, chopped
    - 2 garlic cloves, minced
    - 8 oz mushrooms, chopped
    - 2 cups chopped spinach
    - 1/2 cup shredded mozzarella cheese

  - Instructions:
1. Preheat oven to 375°F (190°C). Grease a baking dish.
2. Season chicken breasts with salt and pepper. Cut a slit in each chicken breast to create a pocket.

3. In a large skillet, heat olive oil over medium heat. Add onion and garlic. Cook until softened, about 5 minutes.

4. Add mushrooms and cook until they release their juices. Stir in spinach and cook until wilted. Remove from heat and let cool slightly.

5. Stuff each chicken breast with the mushroom-spinach mixture. Place in the prepared baking dish.

6. Sprinkle mozzarella cheese over the stuffed chicken breasts.

7. Bake for 25-30 minutes, or until chicken is cooked through.

4. Vegetarian Lentil Moussaka
  - Ingredients:
    - 1 cup dried green lentils
    - 2 cups water
    - 2 tbsp olive oil
    - 1 onion, chopped
    - 2 garlic cloves, minced
    - 1 can (14 oz) diced tomatoes
    - 1 tsp dried oregano
    - 1 tsp ground cinnamon
    - Salt and pepper to taste
    - 2 eggplants, sliced
    - 1 cup Greek yogurt
    - 2 eggs
    - 1/2 cup grated Parmesan cheese

  - Instructions:
    1. Preheat oven to 375°F (190°C). Grease a baking dish.

    2. In a saucepan, combine lentils and water. Bring to a boil, then reduce heat and simmer for 20-25 minutes, or until lentils are tender and water is absorbed.

    3. In a large skillet, heat olive oil over medium heat. Add onion and garlic. Cook until softened, about 5 minutes.

4. Stir in diced tomatoes, oregano, cinnamon, salt, and pepper. Cook for another 5 minutes.

5. In a bowl, whisk together Greek yogurt, eggs, and Parmesan cheese.

6. Layer half of the eggplant slices in the bottom of the prepared baking dish. Top with half of the lentil mixture and half of the yogurt mixture. Repeat layers.

7. Bake for 45-50 minutes, or until the top is golden brown.


5. Sesame Ginger Tofu Stir-Fry
  - Ingredients:
    - 1 block (14 oz) tofu, pressed and cubed
    - 2 tbsp soy sauce
    - 1 tbsp sesame oil
    - 1 tbsp olive oil
    - 2 garlic cloves, minced
    - 1 tbsp grated ginger
    - 1 bell pepper, sliced
    - 1 cup broccoli florets
    - 1 carrot, sliced
    - 2 green onions, sliced
    - 2 tbsp hoisin sauce
    - 1 tbsp rice vinegar
    - 1 tsp honey
    - Sesame seeds for garnish

  - Instructions:
    1. In a bowl, marinate tofu cubes in soy sauce and sesame oil for 15-20 minutes.

    2. In a large skillet, heat olive oil over medium heat. Add garlic and ginger. Cook for 1 minute.

    3. Add marinated tofu to the skillet. Cook until tofu is browned on all sides. Remove from skillet and set aside.

4. In the same skillet, add bell pepper, broccoli, carrot, and green onions. Stir-fry until vegetables are tender-crisp.

5. Return tofu to the skillet. Add hoisin sauce, rice vinegar, and honey. Stir to combine and heat through.

6. Serve hot, garnished with sesame seeds.


6. Quinoa and Black Bean Stuffed Sweet Potatoes
  - Ingredients:
    - 4 sweet potatoes
    - 1 can (14 oz) black beans, drained and rinsed
    - 1 cup cooked quinoa
    - 1 bell pepper, diced
    - 1/2 cup corn kernels
    - 1/2 tsp cumin
    - 1/2 tsp chili powder
    - Salt and pepper to taste
    - Fresh cilantro for garnish
    - Lime wedges for serving

  - Instructions:
    1. Preheat oven to 400°F (200°C). Pierce sweet potatoes with a fork and place on a baking sheet. Bake for 45-60 minutes, or until tender.

    2. In a large bowl, combine black beans, quinoa, bell pepper, corn, cumin, chili powder, salt, and pepper.

    3. Cut a slit in each sweet potato and fluff the flesh with a fork. Spoon the quinoa mixture into each sweet potato.

    4. Garnish with fresh cilantro and serve with lime wedges.


7. Chicken and Vegetable Stir-Fry
  - Ingredients:
    - 1 lb chicken breast, thinly sliced
    - 2 tbsp soy sauce
    - 1 tbsp cornstarch

- 1 tbsp olive oil
- 1 onion, sliced
- 2 bell peppers, sliced
- 1 cup snow peas
- 1 cup broccoli florets
- 2 garlic cloves, minced
- 1 tbsp grated ginger
- 1/4 cup chicken broth
- 2 tbsp hoisin sauce
- 2 green onions, sliced
- Sesame seeds for garnish

- Instructions:
  1. In a bowl, combine chicken slices, soy sauce, and cornstarch. Let marinate for 15-20 minutes.
  2. In a large skillet or wok, heat olive oil over high heat. Add chicken and stir-fry until cooked through. Remove from skillet and set aside.
  3. In the same skillet, add onion, bell peppers, snow peas, broccoli, garlic, and ginger. Stir-fry until vegetables are tender-crisp.
  4. Return chicken to the skillet. Add chicken broth and hoisin sauce. Stir to combine and heat through.
  5. Serve hot, garnished with green onions and sesame seeds.

8. Spaghetti Squash with Turkey Bolognese
  - Ingredients:
    - 1 spaghetti squash
    - 1 lb ground turkey
    - 1 onion, chopped
    - 2 garlic cloves, minced
    - 1 can (14 oz) diced tomatoes
    - 1 can (6 oz) tomato paste
    - 1 tsp dried basil

- 1 tsp dried oregano
- Salt and pepper to taste
- Fresh parsley for garnish

- Instructions:
    1. Preheat oven to 400°F (200°C). Cut spaghetti squash in half lengthwise and scoop out the seeds.
    2. Place spaghetti squash halves cut side down on a baking sheet. Bake for 45-60 minutes, or until tender.
    3. In a large skillet, cook ground turkey over medium heat until browned. Add onion and garlic. Cook until softened, about 5 minutes.
    4. Stir in diced tomatoes, tomato paste, basil, oregano, salt, and pepper. Simmer for 15-20 minutes.
    5. Use a fork to scrape the flesh of the spaghetti squash into strands. Serve topped with turkey Bolognese sauce and garnished with fresh parsley.

9. Shrimp and Vegetable Stir-Fry
  - Ingredients:
    - 1 lb shrimp, peeled and deveined
    - 2 tbsp soy sauce
    - 1 tbsp cornstarch
    - 1 tbsp olive oil
    - 1 onion, sliced
    - 2 bell peppers, sliced
    - 1 cup snap peas
    - 1 cup sliced mushrooms
    - 2 garlic cloves, minced
    - 1 tbsp grated ginger
    - 1/4 cup chicken broth
    - 2 tbsp hoisin sauce
    - 2 green onions, sliced
    - Sesame seeds for garnish

- Instructions:

1. In a bowl, combine shrimp, soy sauce, and cornstarch. Let marinate for 15-20 minutes.

2. In a large skillet or wok, heat olive oil over high heat. Add shrimp and stir-fry until pink and opaque. Remove from skillet and set aside.

3. In the same skillet, add onion, bell peppers, snap peas, mushrooms, garlic, and ginger. Stir-fry until vegetables are tender-crisp.

4. Return shrimp to the skillet. Add chicken broth and hoisin sauce. Stir to combine and heat through.

5. Serve hot, garnished with green onions and sesame seeds.

10. Eggplant Parmesan
   - Ingredients:
     - 2 eggplants, sliced
     - Salt
     - 2 cups marinara sauce
     - 1 cup shredded mozzarella cheese
     - 1/2 cup grated Parmesan cheese
     - 1/4 cup chopped fresh basil

   - Instructions:

1. Preheat oven to 375°F (190°C). Grease a baking dish.

2. Place eggplant slices on a baking sheet and sprinkle with salt. Let sit for 20 minutes, then pat dry with paper towels.

3. Arrange a layer of eggplant slices in the bottom of the prepared baking dish. Top with marinara sauce, mozzarella cheese, Parmesan cheese, and basil. Repeat layers.

4. Cover with foil and bake for 30 minutes. Remove foil and bake for an additional 15 minutes, or until cheese is melted and bubbly.

11. Coconut Curry Lentil Soup
  - Ingredients:
    - 1 cup red lentils
    - 4 cups vegetable broth
    - 1 can (14 oz) coconut milk
    - 1 onion, chopped
    - 2 garlic cloves, minced
    - 1 tbsp curry powder
    - 1 tsp ground cumin
    - 1 tsp ground turmeric
    - 1 tsp ground ginger
    - Salt and pepper to taste
    - Fresh cilantro for garnish

  - Instructions:
    1. In a large pot, combine lentils and vegetable broth. Bring to a boil, then reduce heat and simmer for 15-20 minutes, or until lentils are tender.
    2. In a skillet, heat olive oil over medium heat. Add onion and garlic. Cook until softened, about 5 minutes.
    3. Stir in curry powder, cumin, turmeric, ginger, salt, and pepper. Cook for another minute.
    4. Add spiced onion mixture to the pot of lentils. Stir in coconut milk. Simmer for another 5-10 minutes.
    5. Serve hot, garnished with fresh cilantro.

12. Vegetable Stir-Fry with Brown Rice
  - Ingredients:
    - 2 cups cooked brown rice
    - 2 tbsp soy sauce
    - 1 tbsp sesame oil
    - 1 tbsp olive oil
    - 1 onion, sliced

- 2 garlic cloves, minced
- 1 bell pepper, sliced
- 1 zucchini, sliced
- 1 cup broccoli florets
- 1 cup sliced mushrooms
- Salt and pepper to taste
- Sesame seeds for garnish

- Instructions:
1. In a large skillet, heat olive oil over medium heat. Add onion and garlic. Cook until softened, about 5 minutes.
2. Add bell pepper, zucchini, broccoli, and mushrooms. Stir-fry until vegetables are tender-crisp.
3. Stir in cooked brown rice, soy sauce, sesame oil, salt, and pepper. Cook for another 2-3 minutes.
4. Serve hot, garnished with sesame seeds.

13. Baked Stuffed Portobello Mushrooms
  - Ingredients:
    - 4 large portobello mushrooms, stems removed
    - 2 tbsp olive oil
    - 2 garlic cloves, minced
    - 1/2 onion, chopped
    - 1/2 cup chopped bell pepper
    - 1/2 cup chopped spinach
    - 1/2 cup breadcrumbs
    - 1/4 cup grated Parmesan cheese
    - Salt and pepper to taste
    - Fresh parsley for garnish

- Instructions:
1. Preheat oven to 400°F (200°C). Grease a baking dish.

2. Place portobello mushrooms in the prepared baking dish, gill side up.

3. In a skillet, heat olive oil over medium heat. Add garlic, onion, and bell pepper. Cook until softened, about 5 minutes.

4. Stir in spinach, breadcrumbs, Parmesan cheese, salt, and pepper. Cook for another 2-3 minutes.

5. Spoon the breadcrumb mixture into the portobello mushrooms.

6. Bake for 20-25 minutes, or until mushrooms are tender.

7. Serve hot, garnished with fresh parsley.

14. Chickpea and Spinach Curry
  - Ingredients:
    - 1 can (14 oz) chickpeas, drained and rinsed
    - 2 tbsp olive oil
    - 1 onion, chopped
    - 2 garlic cloves, minced
    - 1 tbsp curry powder
    - 1 tsp ground cumin
    - 1 tsp ground coriander
    - 1/2 tsp turmeric
    - 1 can (14 oz) diced tomatoes
    - 1 can (14 oz) coconut milk
    - 2 cups chopped spinach
    - Salt and pepper to taste

  - Instructions:
    1. In a large skillet, heat olive oil over medium heat. Add onion and garlic. Cook until softened, about 5 minutes.

    2. Stir in curry powder, cumin, coriander, and turmeric. Cook for another minute.

    3. Add chickpeas, diced tomatoes, and coconut milk. Simmer for 10-15 minutes.

    4. Stir in chopped spinach and cook until wilted.

5. Serve hot, over cooked brown rice or quinoa.

15. Sweet Potato and Black Bean Enchiladas
   - Ingredients:
     - 2 sweet potatoes, peeled and diced
     - 1 can (14 oz) black beans, drained and rinsed
     - 1 onion, chopped
     - 2 garlic cloves, minced
     - 1 bell pepper, chopped
     - 1 can (14 oz) enchilada sauce
     - 8 whole wheat tortillas
     - 1/2 cup shredded cheddar cheese
     - Fresh cilantro for garnish

   - Instructions:
     1. Preheat oven to 375°F (190°C). Grease a baking dish.
     2. Steam sweet potatoes until tender, about 15 minutes.
     3. In a skillet, heat olive oil over medium heat. Add onion, garlic, and bell pepper. Cook until softened, about 5 minutes.
     4. Stir in cooked sweet potatoes and black beans.
     5. Spread a thin layer of enchilada sauce on the bottom of the prepared baking dish.
     6. Fill each tortilla with the sweet potato-black bean mixture. Roll up and place seam-side down in the baking dish.
     7. Pour remaining enchilada sauce over the top. Sprinkle with shredded cheddar cheese.
     8. Bake for 20-25 minutes, or until cheese is melted and bubbly.
     9. Serve hot, garnished with fresh cilantro.

16. Vegetable Coconut Curry
   - Ingredients:
     - 1 tbsp olive oil
     - 1 onion, chopped

- 2 garlic cloves, minced
- 1 tbsp curry powder
- 1 tsp ground turmeric
- 1 tsp ground cumin
- 1 can (14 oz) coconut milk
- 1 cup vegetable broth
- 2 carrots, sliced
- 1 bell pepper, chopped
- 1 zucchini, chopped
- 1 cup chopped spinach
- Salt and pepper to taste
- Cooked rice for serving

- Instructions:
    1. In a large skillet, heat olive oil over medium heat. Add onion and garlic. Cook until softened, about 5 minutes.
    2. Stir in curry powder, turmeric, and cumin. Cook for another minute.
    3. Add coconut milk and vegetable broth. Bring to a simmer.
    4. Add carrots, bell pepper, and zucchini. Simmer for 10-15 minutes, or until vegetables are tender.
    5. Stir in chopped spinach and cook until wilted.
    6. Season with salt and pepper. Serve hot over cooked rice.

17. Lemon Garlic Shrimp with Quinoa
   - Ingredients:
    - 1 cup quinoa
    - 2 cups water
    - 1 lb shrimp, peeled and deveined
    - Salt and pepper to taste
    - 2 tbsp olive oil
    - 4 garlic cloves, minced
    - Zest and juice of 1 lemon

- 2 tbsp chopped fresh parsley

  - Instructions:
    1. Rinse quinoa under cold water. In a saucepan, combine quinoa and water. Bring to a boil, then reduce heat and simmer for 15-20 minutes, or until quinoa is tender and water is absorbed.
    2. Season shrimp with salt and pepper. In a large skillet, heat olive oil over medium heat. Add shrimp and cook until pink and opaque, about 2-3 minutes per side. Remove shrimp from skillet and set aside.
    3. In the same skillet, add garlic and cook for 1 minute. Stir in lemon zest and juice.
    4. Return shrimp to the skillet and toss to coat in the lemon garlic sauce.
    5. Serve hot over cooked quinoa, garnished with chopped parsley.

18. Cauliflower Rice Stir-Fry
  - Ingredients:
    - 1 head cauliflower, grated into rice-like pieces
    - 2 tbsp sesame oil
    - 1 onion, chopped
    - 2 garlic cloves, minced
    - 1 bell pepper, chopped
    - 1 zucchini, chopped
    - 1 cup chopped broccoli
    - 2 tbsp soy sauce
    - 1 tsp sriracha sauce (optional)
    - Salt and pepper to taste
    - Sesame seeds for garnish

  - Instructions:
    1. In a large skillet, heat sesame oil over medium heat. Add onion and garlic. Cook until softened, about 5 minutes.

2. Add bell pepper, zucchini, broccoli, and cauliflower rice. Stir-fry until vegetables are tender-crisp.

3. Stir in soy sauce, sriracha sauce, salt, and pepper.

4. Serve hot, garnished with sesame seeds.


19. Butternut Squash and Black Bean Tacos
  - Ingredients:
    - 2 cups diced butternut squash
    - 1 tbsp olive oil
    - 1 tsp chili powder
    - 1/2 tsp ground cumin
    - Salt and pepper to taste
    - 1 can (14 oz) black beans, drained and rinsed
    - 8 small corn tortillas
    - 1/2 cup diced tomatoes
    - 1/4 cup chopped fresh cilantro
    - Lime wedges for serving

  - Instructions:
    1. Preheat oven to 400°F (200°C). Line a baking sheet with parchment paper.

    2. In a bowl, toss butternut squash with olive oil, chili powder, cumin, salt, and pepper. Spread on the prepared baking sheet.

    3. Roast squash for 20-25 minutes, or until tender.

    4. In a skillet, heat black beans over medium heat until heated through.

    5. Warm tortillas in a dry skillet over medium heat.

    6. Assemble tacos with roasted butternut squash, black beans, diced tomatoes, and chopped cilantro.

    7. Serve with lime wedges for squeezing.


20. Spinach and Mushroom Stuffed Spaghetti Squash
  - Ingredients:

- 1 spaghetti squash, halved and seeded
- 1 tbsp olive oil
- 1 onion, chopped
- 2 garlic cloves, minced
- 8 oz mushrooms, chopped
- 4 cups chopped spinach
- 1/2 cup grated Parmesan cheese
- Salt and pepper to taste

- Instructions:

1. Preheat oven to 400°F (200°C). Place spaghetti squash halves cut-side down on a baking sheet. Bake for 30-40 minutes, or until tender.

2. In a large skillet, heat olive oil over medium heat. Add onion and garlic. Cook until softened, about 5 minutes.

3. Add mushrooms and cook until they release their juices. Stir in chopped spinach and cook until wilted.

4. Use a fork to scrape the spaghetti squash flesh into strands. Add the vegetable mixture to the spaghetti squash strands. Stir in Parmesan cheese.

5. Season with salt and pepper. Serve hot.

# Chapter 4: Sides and Snacks for Energy

1. Turmeric Roasted Cauliflower
   - Ingredients:
     - 1 head cauliflower, cut into florets
     - 2 tbsp olive oil
     - 1 tsp turmeric
     - 1/2 tsp cumin
     - 1/2 tsp smoked paprika
     - Salt and pepper to taste
     - Fresh parsley for garnish

   - Instructions:
     1. Preheat oven to 425°F (220°C). Line a baking sheet with parchment paper.
     2. In a large bowl, toss cauliflower florets with olive oil, turmeric, cumin, smoked paprika, salt, and pepper.
     3. Spread cauliflower in a single layer on the prepared baking sheet.
     4. Roast for 20-25 minutes, or until cauliflower is tender and golden brown.
     5. Garnish with fresh parsley before serving.

2. Quinoa Salad with Chickpeas and Lemon Dressing
   - Ingredients:
     - 1 cup cooked quinoa
     - 1 can (14 oz) chickpeas, drained and rinsed
     - 1 cucumber, diced
     - 1 bell pepper, diced
     - 1/4 cup chopped fresh parsley
     - 1/4 cup olive oil
     - Zest and juice of 1 lemon
     - 1 garlic clove, minced
     - Salt and pepper to taste

- Instructions:
    1. In a large bowl, combine cooked quinoa, chickpeas, cucumber, bell pepper, and parsley.
    2. In a small bowl, whisk together olive oil, lemon zest, lemon juice, garlic, salt, and pepper.
    3. Pour dressing over the quinoa mixture and toss to combine.
    4. Serve chilled or at room temperature.

3. Sweet Potato Hummus with Veggie Sticks
  - Ingredients:
    - 1 can (14 oz) chickpeas, drained and rinsed
    - 1 sweet potato, peeled, cooked, and mashed
    - 2 tbsp tahini
    - 2 tbsp olive oil
    - 1 garlic clove, minced
    - Juice of 1 lemon
    - Salt and pepper to taste
    - Assorted veggie sticks (carrots, celery, bell peppers) for serving

  - Instructions:
    1. In a food processor, combine chickpeas, mashed sweet potato, tahini, olive oil, garlic, lemon juice, salt, and pepper.
    2. Process until smooth and creamy, adding water as needed to reach desired consistency.
    3. Serve sweet potato hummus with veggie sticks.

4. Baked Kale Chips
  - Ingredients:
    - 1 bunch kale, stems removed and leaves torn into bite-sized pieces
    - 1 tbsp olive oil
    - Salt and pepper to taste

- Instructions:
   1. Preheat oven to 350°F (175°C). Line a baking sheet with parchment paper.
   2. In a large bowl, toss kale leaves with olive oil, salt, and pepper.
   3. Spread kale in a single layer on the prepared baking sheet.
   4. Bake for 10-15 minutes, or until kale is crispy.
   5. Let cool before serving.

5. Chia Seed Pudding
   - Ingredients:
     - 1/4 cup chia seeds
     - 1 cup unsweetened almond milk
     - 1 tbsp maple syrup
     - 1/2 tsp vanilla extract
     - Fresh berries for topping

   - Instructions:
     1. In a bowl, combine chia seeds, almond milk, maple syrup, and vanilla extract. Stir well.
     2. Cover and refrigerate for at least 2 hours, or overnight, until thickened.
     3. Serve chilled, topped with fresh berries.

6. Roasted Beet and Carrot Salad
   - Ingredients:
     - 2 beets, peeled and diced
     - 2 carrots, peeled and diced
     - 2 tbsp olive oil
     - 1 tsp cumin
     - 1/2 tsp smoked paprika
     - Salt and pepper to taste
     - 2 cups mixed greens
     - 1/4 cup crumbled feta cheese

- 2 tbsp balsamic glaze

- Instructions:
    1. Preheat oven to 400°F (200°C). Line a baking sheet with parchment paper.
    2. In a bowl, toss diced beets and carrots with olive oil, cumin, smoked paprika, salt, and pepper.
    3. Spread vegetables in a single layer on the prepared baking sheet.
    4. Roast for 25-30 minutes, or until vegetables are tender and caramelized.
    5. Serve roasted beets and carrots over mixed greens, topped with crumbled feta cheese and balsamic glaze.

7. Spiced Almonds
  - Ingredients:
    - 1 cup raw almonds
    - 1 tbsp olive oil
    - 1 tsp smoked paprika
    - 1/2 tsp cumin
    - 1/2 tsp garlic powder
    - 1/2 tsp onion powder
    - 1/2 tsp sea salt

  - Instructions:
    1. Preheat oven to 350°F (175°C). Line a baking sheet with parchment paper.
    2. In a bowl, toss almonds with olive oil, smoked paprika, cumin, garlic powder, onion powder, and sea salt.
    3. Spread almonds in a single layer on the prepared baking sheet.
    4. Bake for 10-15 minutes, stirring halfway through, until almonds are toasted.
    5. Let cool before serving.

8. Cucumber Avocado Salsa
  - Ingredients:
    - 1 cucumber, diced
    - 1 avocado, diced
    - 1/4 cup diced red onion
    - 1/4 cup chopped fresh cilantro
    - Juice of 1 lime
    - Salt and pepper to taste
    - Tortilla chips for serving

  - Instructions:
    1. In a bowl, combine diced cucumber, diced avocado, red onion, cilantro, lime juice, salt, and pepper. Stir gently to combine.
    2. Serve cucumber avocado salsa with tortilla chips.

9. Hummus-Stuffed Mini Peppers
  - Ingredients:
    - 12 mini bell peppers, halved and seeded
    - 1 cup hummus
    - Fresh parsley for garnish

  - Instructions:
    1. Fill each mini pepper half with a spoonful of hummus.
    2. Garnish with fresh parsley before serving.

10. Roasted Red Pepper and Walnut Dip
  - Ingredients:
    - 1 cup roasted red peppers (from a jar), drained
    - 1/2 cup walnuts
    - 2 tbsp olive oil
    - 1 tbsp lemon juice
    - 1 garlic clove
    - Salt and pepper to taste

- Pita bread or vegetable sticks for serving

  - Instructions:
    1. In a food processor, combine roasted red peppers, walnuts, olive oil, lemon juice, garlic, salt, and pepper.
    2. Process until smooth and creamy.
    3. Serve roasted red pepper and walnut dip with pita bread or vegetable sticks.

11. Edamame and Mint Salad
    - Ingredients:
      - 2 cups shelled edamame, cooked
      - 1/4 cup chopped fresh mint
      - 1/4 cup chopped red onion
      - 2 tbsp olive oil
      - 1 tbsp lemon juice
      - Salt and pepper to taste

  - Instructions:
    1. In a bowl, combine cooked edamame, chopped mint, chopped red onion, olive oil, lemon juice, salt, and pepper. Stir to combine.
    2. Serve chilled or at room temperature.

12. Baked Sweet Potato Fries
    - Ingredients:
      - 2 sweet potatoes, cut into fries
      - 2 tbsp olive oil
      - 1 tsp smoked paprika
      - 1/2 tsp garlic powder
      - 1/2 tsp onion powder
      - Salt and pepper to taste

  - Instructions:

1. Preheat oven to 425°F (220°C). Line a baking sheet with parchment paper.

2. In a bowl, toss sweet potato fries with olive oil, smoked paprika, garlic powder, onion powder, salt, and pepper.

3. Spread fries in a single layer on the prepared baking sheet.

4. Bake for 20-25 minutes, flipping halfway through, until fries are crispy and golden brown.

5. Serve hot.

13. Greek Yogurt Parfait with Berries and Almonds
   - Ingredients:
   - 1 cup Greek yogurt
      - 1/2 cup mixed berries (such as strawberries, blueberries, raspberries)
   - 2 tbsp sliced almonds
   - 1 tbsp honey

   - Instructions:
   1. In a glass, layer Greek yogurt, mixed berries, sliced almonds, and honey.

2. Repeat layers if desired.

3. Serve chilled.

14. Roasted Garlic and White Bean Dip
   - Ingredients:
   - 1 can (14 oz) white beans, drained and rinsed
   - 2 tbsp olive oil
   - 2 garlic cloves, roasted
   - 1 tbsp lemon juice
   - Salt and pepper to taste
   - Fresh parsley for garnish

   - Instructions:

1. In a food processor, combine white beans, olive oil, roasted garlic cloves, lemon juice, salt, and pepper.

2. Process until smooth and creamy.

3. Serve roasted garlic and white bean dip garnished with fresh parsley.

15. Chia Seed Energy Balls
   - Ingredients:
     - 1/2 cup dates, pitted
     - 1/2 cup almonds
     - 2 tbsp chia seeds
     - 2 tbsp unsweetened cocoa powder
     - 1/2 tsp vanilla extract
     - Pinch of salt
     - Water, as needed

   - Instructions:
     1. In a food processor, combine dates, almonds, chia seeds, cocoa powder, vanilla extract, and salt.

     2. Process until mixture starts to come together. Add water, 1 tablespoon at a time, if needed.

     3. Roll mixture into small balls.

     4. Refrigerate for at least 30 minutes before serving.

16. Roasted Brussels Sprouts with Balsamic Glaze
   - Ingredients:
     - 1 lb Brussels sprouts, trimmed and halved
     - 2 tbsp olive oil
     - Salt and pepper to taste
     - Balsamic glaze for drizzling

   - Instructions:

1. Preheat oven to 400°F (200°C). Line a baking sheet with parchment paper.

2. In a bowl, toss Brussels sprouts with olive oil, salt, and pepper.

3. Spread Brussels sprouts in a single layer on the prepared baking sheet.

4. Roast for 20-25 minutes, or until Brussels sprouts are tender and caramelized.

5. Drizzle with balsamic glaze before serving.

17. Almond Butter Banana Bites
  - Ingredients:
    - 2 bananas, peeled and sliced
    - 2 tbsp almond butter
    - 2 tbsp granola

  - Instructions:
    1. Spread almond butter on banana slices.
    2. Sprinkle with granola.
    3. Serve as a healthy snack.

18. Roasted Chickpeas
  - Ingredients:
    - 1 can (14 oz) chickpeas, drained and rinsed
    - 1 tbsp olive oil
    - 1 tsp smoked paprika
    - 1/2 tsp cumin
    - 1/2 tsp garlic powder
    - Salt and pepper to taste

  - Instructions:
    1. Preheat oven to 400°F (200°C). Line a baking sheet with parchment paper.

2. In a bowl, toss chickpeas with olive oil, smoked paprika, cumin, garlic powder, salt, and pepper.

3. Spread chickpeas in a single layer on the prepared baking sheet.

4. Roast for 20-25 minutes, shaking the pan halfway through, until chickpeas are crispy.

5. Let cool before serving.

19. Stuffed Mini Bell Peppers
   - Ingredients:
     - 12 mini bell peppers, halved and seeded
     - 1/2 cup whipped cream cheese
     - 1/4 cup chopped fresh chives
     - Salt and pepper to taste

   - Instructions:
     1. Fill each mini pepper half with a spoonful of whipped cream cheese.

2. Sprinkle with chopped chives, salt, and pepper.

3. Serve as a tasty appetizer or snack.

20. Apple Cinnamon Oat Bars
   - Ingredients:
     - 2 cups rolled oats
     - 1/2 cup unsweetened applesauce
     - 1/4 cup maple syrup
     - 1 tsp cinnamon
     - 1/2 tsp vanilla extract
     - Pinch of salt
     - 1/2 cup chopped dried apples

   - Instructions:
   1. Preheat oven to 350°F (175°C). Grease a baking dish.

2. In a bowl, combine rolled oats, applesauce, maple syrup, cinnamon, vanilla extract, salt, and chopped dried apples.

3. Press mixture into the prepared baking dish.

4. Bake for 30-35 minutes, or until golden brown.

5. Let cool before cutting into bars.

# Chapter 5: Comforting Dinners

1. Slow Cooker Chicken and Vegetable Stew
   - Ingredients:
     - 1 lb boneless, skinless chicken thighs
     - 4 carrots, peeled and sliced
     - 2 celery stalks, sliced
     - 1 onion, chopped
     - 2 garlic cloves, minced
     - 4 cups chicken broth
     - 1 can (14 oz) diced tomatoes
     - 1 tsp dried thyme
     - 1 tsp dried rosemary
     - Salt and pepper to taste
     - Fresh parsley for garnish

   - Instructions:
     1. Place chicken thighs, carrots, celery, onion, garlic, chicken broth, diced tomatoes, thyme, rosemary, salt, and pepper in a slow cooker.
     2. Cover and cook on low for 6-8 hours or high for 3-4 hours, until chicken is tender.
     3. Remove chicken from the slow cooker and shred with two forks. Return chicken to the slow cooker and stir to combine.
     4. Serve hot, garnished with fresh parsley.

2. Vegetable and Lentil Shepherd's Pie
   - Ingredients:
     - 1 cup dry green or brown lentils
     - 2 cups vegetable broth
     - 2 tbsp olive oil
     - 1 onion, chopped
     - 2 carrots, diced
     - 2 celery stalks, diced

- 2 garlic cloves, minced
- 1 tsp dried thyme
- 1 tsp dried rosemary
- Salt and pepper to taste
- 4 cups mashed potatoes
- Fresh parsley for garnish

- Instructions:
1. Preheat oven to 375°F (190°C). Grease a baking dish.
2. In a saucepan, combine lentils and vegetable broth. Bring to a boil, then reduce heat and simmer for 20-25 minutes, until lentils are tender.
3. In a large skillet, heat olive oil over medium heat. Add onion, carrots, celery, and garlic. Cook until vegetables are softened, about 5-7 minutes.
4. Stir in cooked lentils, dried thyme, dried rosemary, salt, and pepper. Cook for another 5 minutes.
5. Transfer lentil mixture to the prepared baking dish. Spread mashed potatoes over the top.
6. Bake for 25-30 minutes, or until heated through and potatoes are golden brown.
7. Serve hot, garnished with fresh parsley.

3. One-Pot Chicken and Rice Casserole
  - Ingredients:
  - 1 lb boneless, skinless chicken breasts, cut into bite-sized pieces
  - 1 onion, chopped
  - 2 garlic cloves, minced
  - 1 bell pepper, chopped
  - 1 cup long-grain white rice
  - 2 cups chicken broth
  - 1 can (14 oz) diced tomatoes
  - 1 tsp paprika

- 1/2 tsp dried oregano
- Salt and pepper to taste
- Fresh parsley for garnish

- Instructions:
1. In a large skillet or pot, heat olive oil over medium-high heat. Add chicken and cook until browned, about 5 minutes.
2. Add onion, garlic, and bell pepper. Cook until vegetables are softened, about 5 minutes.
3. Stir in rice, chicken broth, diced tomatoes, paprika, oregano, salt, and pepper. Bring to a boil, then reduce heat and simmer for 20-25 minutes, until rice is cooked through.
4. Serve hot, garnished with fresh parsley.

4. Baked Salmon with Lemon and Dill
   - Ingredients:
     - 4 salmon fillets
     - 2 tbsp olive oil
     - 2 tbsp lemon juice
     - 2 garlic cloves, minced
     - 1 tbsp chopped fresh dill
     - Salt and pepper to taste
     - Lemon slices for garnish

   - Instructions:
1. Preheat oven to 400°F (200°C). Grease a baking dish.
2. Place salmon fillets in the baking dish.
3. In a small bowl, whisk together olive oil, lemon juice, minced garlic, chopped dill, salt, and pepper.
4. Pour the mixture over the salmon fillets, making sure they are evenly coated.
5. Bake for 12-15 minutes, or until salmon is cooked through and flakes easily with a fork.

6. Serve hot, garnished with lemon slices.

5. Creamy Mushroom and Spinach Pasta
   - Ingredients:
     - 8 oz pasta of your choice
     - 2 tbsp olive oil
     - 8 oz mushrooms, sliced
     - 2 garlic cloves, minced
     - 4 cups fresh spinach
     - 1 cup heavy cream
     - 1/2 cup grated Parmesan cheese
     - Salt and pepper to taste
     - Fresh parsley for garnish

   - Instructions:
     1. Cook pasta according to package instructions. Drain and set aside.
     2. In a large skillet, heat olive oil over medium heat. Add mushrooms and cook until browned, about 5 minutes.
     3. Add minced garlic and cook for another minute.
     4. Stir in fresh spinach and cook until wilted.
     5. Reduce heat to low and stir in heavy cream and grated Parmesan cheese. Cook until heated through and slightly thickened.
     6. Season with salt and pepper to taste. Add cooked pasta to the skillet and toss to combine.
     7. Serve hot, garnished with fresh parsley.

6. Roasted Vegetable Quinoa Bowls
   - Ingredients:
     - 1 cup quinoa, cooked
     - 1 sweet potato, peeled and diced
     - 1 zucchini, diced
     - 1 red bell pepper, diced

- 1 onion, chopped
- 2 tbsp olive oil
- 1 tsp smoked paprika
- 1/2 tsp garlic powder
- Salt and pepper to taste
- 1/4 cup crumbled feta cheese
- Fresh parsley for garnish

- Instructions:
   1. Preheat oven to 425°F (220°C). Line a baking sheet with parchment paper.
   2. In a bowl, toss diced sweet potato, zucchini, red bell pepper, and onion with olive oil, smoked paprika, garlic powder, salt, and pepper.
   3. Spread vegetables in a single layer on the prepared baking sheet.
   4. Roast for 25-30 minutes, or until vegetables are tender and caramelized.
   5. Divide cooked quinoa among bowls. Top with roasted vegetables, crumbled feta cheese, and fresh parsley.
   6. Serve hot.

7. Turkey and Vegetable Stir-Fry
   - Ingredients:
     - 1 lb turkey breast, sliced into strips
     - 2 tbsp soy sauce
     - 1 tbsp hoisin sauce
     - 1 tbsp rice vinegar
     - 1 tbsp sesame oil
     - 1 onion, sliced
     - 1 bell pepper, sliced
     - 1 zucchini, sliced
     - 1 cup broccoli florets
     - 2 garlic cloves, minced
     - Cooked brown rice for serving

- Instructions:

1. In a bowl, combine sliced turkey breast with soy sauce, hoisin sauce, rice vinegar, and sesame oil. Marinate for 15-30 minutes.

2. In a large skillet or wok, heat olive oil over medium-high heat. Add marinated turkey and cook until browned and cooked through, about 5-7 minutes. Remove from skillet and set aside.

3. In the same skillet, add onion, bell pepper, zucchini, broccoli, and minced garlic. Stir-fry until vegetables are tender-crisp, about 5 minutes.

4. Return cooked turkey to the skillet and toss to combine.

5. Serve hot over cooked brown rice.


8. Mushroom and Spinach Risotto
  - Ingredients:
    - 2 tbsp olive oil
    - 1 onion, chopped
    - 2 garlic cloves, minced
    - 8 oz mushrooms, sliced
    - 2 cups Arborio rice
    - 1/2 cup dry white wine (optional)
    - 6 cups vegetable broth, warmed
    - 4 cups baby spinach
    - 1/2 cup grated Parmesan cheese
    - Salt and pepper to taste

  - Instructions:

1. In a large skillet or pot, heat olive oil over medium heat. Add onion and garlic, cook until softened, about 5 minutes.

2. Add sliced mushrooms and cook until browned and tender, about 5-7 minutes.

3. Stir in Arborio rice and cook for 2 minutes, stirring constantly.

4. If using, pour in white wine and cook until absorbed, stirring occasionally.

5. Gradually add warmed vegetable broth, 1 cup at a time, stirring frequently until absorbed before adding more.

6. Continue cooking and stirring until rice is creamy and tender, about 20-25 minutes.

7. Stir in baby spinach and grated Parmesan cheese until spinach is wilted and cheese is melted.

8. Season with salt and pepper to taste. Serve hot.

9. Spaghetti Squash with Bolognese Sauce
  - Ingredients:
    - 1 spaghetti squash, halved and seeds removed
    - 1 lb ground beef
    - 1 onion, chopped
    - 2 garlic cloves, minced
    - 1 can (14 oz) crushed tomatoes
    - 1 tsp dried oregano
    - 1 tsp dried basil
    - Salt and pepper to taste
    - Fresh parsley for garnish
    - Grated Parmesan cheese for serving

  - Instructions:
    1. Preheat oven to 400°F (200°C). Place spaghetti squash halves cut side down on a baking sheet. Bake for 30-40 minutes, or until tender.

    2. In a large skillet, cook ground beef over medium-high heat until browned. Add chopped onion and minced garlic, cook for another 5 minutes.

    3. Stir in crushed tomatoes, dried oregano, dried basil, salt, and pepper. Simmer for 10-15 minutes.

4. Scrape the spaghetti squash flesh with a fork to create "noodles." Serve with Bolognese sauce on top. Garnish with fresh parsley and grated Parmesan cheese.

10. Chicken and Vegetable Stir-Fry
   - Ingredients:
    - 1 lb boneless, skinless chicken breasts, cut into strips
    - 2 tbsp soy sauce
    - 1 tbsp sesame oil
    - 2 garlic cloves, minced
    - 1 tsp ginger, minced
    - 1 onion, sliced
    - 1 bell pepper, sliced
    - 1 cup broccoli florets
    - 1 cup snap peas
    - Cooked rice for serving

   - Instructions:
    1. In a bowl, marinate chicken strips in soy sauce and sesame oil for 30 minutes.
    2. Heat olive oil in a large skillet or wok over medium-high heat. Add minced garlic and ginger, cook for 1 minute.
    3. Add marinated chicken strips and cook until browned and cooked through, about 5-7 minutes.
    4. Add sliced onion, bell pepper, broccoli florets, and snap peas. Stir-fry for another 5-7 minutes, until vegetables are tender-crisp.
    5. Serve chicken and vegetable stir-fry over cooked rice.

11. Vegan Lentil Curry
   - Ingredients:
    - 1 cup dry red lentils
    - 4 cups vegetable broth
    - 1 onion, chopped

- 2 garlic cloves, minced
- 1 tbsp curry powder
- 1 tsp ground cumin
- 1 can (14 oz) coconut milk
- Salt and pepper to taste
- Fresh cilantro for garnish

- Instructions:
1. In a large pot, combine red lentils and vegetable broth. Bring to a boil, then reduce heat and simmer for 20-25 minutes, until lentils are tender.
2. In a separate skillet, heat olive oil over medium heat. Add chopped onion and minced garlic, cook until softened, about 5 minutes.
3. Stir in curry powder and ground cumin. Cook for another minute.
4. Add cooked lentils and coconut milk to the skillet. Season with salt and pepper. Simmer for 10 minutes.
5. Serve hot, garnished with fresh cilantro.

12. Spinach and Ricotta Stuffed Shells
  - Ingredients:
    - 1 box (12 oz) jumbo pasta shells
    - 2 cups ricotta cheese
    - 1 cup grated Parmesan cheese
    - 1 egg, beaten
    - 1 cup chopped spinach, cooked and drained
    - 2 cups marinara sauce
    - 1 cup shredded mozzarella cheese
    - Fresh basil for garnish

  - Instructions:
    1. Preheat oven to 375°F (190°C). Cook jumbo pasta shells according to package instructions. Drain and set aside.

2. In a bowl, combine ricotta cheese, grated Parmesan cheese, beaten egg, and chopped spinach.

3. Stuff cooked pasta shells with the ricotta mixture and place them in a baking dish.

4. Pour marinara sauce over the stuffed shells. Sprinkle with shredded mozzarella cheese.

5. Cover with foil and bake for 25-30 minutes, or until cheese is melted and bubbly.

6. Serve hot, garnished with fresh basil.

13. Beef and Vegetable Stew
  - Ingredients:
    - 1 lb stewing beef, cubed
    - 2 tbsp olive oil
    - 1 onion, chopped
    - 2 garlic cloves, minced
    - 2 carrots, diced
    - 2 celery stalks, diced
    - 2 potatoes, peeled and diced
    - 4 cups beef broth
    - 1 can (14 oz) diced tomatoes
    - 1 tsp dried thyme
    - 1 tsp dried rosemary
    - Salt and pepper to taste
    - Fresh parsley for garnish

  - Instructions:
    1. In a large pot, heat olive oil over medium-high heat. Add cubed stewing beef and cook until browned on all sides.

    2. Add chopped onion and minced garlic, cook until softened, about 5 minutes.

    3. Stir in diced carrots, celery, potatoes, beef broth, diced tomatoes, dried thyme, dried rosemary, salt, and pepper.

4. Bring to a boil, then reduce heat and simmer for 1-2 hours, until beef is tender.

5. Serve hot, garnished with fresh parsley.

14. Baked Chicken Parmesan
  - Ingredients:
    - 4 boneless, skinless chicken breasts
    - Salt and pepper to taste
    - 1 cup breadcrumbs
    - 1/2 cup grated Parmesan cheese
    - 1 tsp dried oregano
    - 1 tsp dried basil
    - 1 egg, beaten
    - 1 cup marinara sauce
    - 1 cup shredded mozzarella cheese
    - Fresh basil for garnish

  - Instructions:
    1. Preheat oven to 400°F (200°C). Grease a baking dish.

    2. Season chicken breasts with salt and pepper.

    3. In a shallow dish, combine breadcrumbs, grated Parmesan cheese, dried oregano, and dried basil.

    4. Dip each chicken breast in beaten egg, then coat with breadcrumb mixture.

    5. Place coated chicken breasts in the prepared baking dish. Bake for 20-25 minutes, or until chicken is cooked through.

    6. Spoon marinara sauce over the chicken breasts and sprinkle with shredded mozzarella cheese.

    7. Bake for another 5-10 minutes, or until cheese is melted and bubbly.

    8. Serve hot, garnished with fresh basil.

15. Vegetarian Chili

- Ingredients:
  - 1 tbsp olive oil
  - 1 onion, chopped
  -- 2 garlic cloves, minced
  - 1 bell pepper, chopped
  - 1 zucchini, diced
  - 1 carrot, diced
  - 1 can (14 oz) diced tomatoes
  - 1 can (14 oz) black beans, drained and rinsed
  - 1 can (14 oz) kidney beans, drained and rinsed
  - 2 cups vegetable broth
  - 2 tsp chili powder
  - 1 tsp cumin
  - 1/2 tsp paprika
  - Salt and pepper to taste
  - Optional toppings: chopped cilantro, sliced avocado, shredded cheese, sour cream

- Instructions:
  1. In a large pot, heat olive oil over medium heat. Add onion and garlic, cook until softened, about 5 minutes.
  2. Add bell pepper, zucchini, and carrot. Cook for another 5 minutes.
  3. Stir in diced tomatoes, black beans, kidney beans, vegetable broth, chili powder, cumin, paprika, salt, and pepper. Bring to a simmer.
  4. Simmer uncovered for 20-25 minutes, stirring occasionally.
  5. Serve hot, garnished with optional toppings if desired.

16. Veggie-Packed Macaroni and Cheese
  - Ingredients:
  - 8 oz elbow macaroni

- 2 tbsp butter
- 2 tbsp all-purpose flour
- 2 cups milk
- 2 cups shredded cheddar cheese
- 1 cup diced bell peppers
- 1 cup diced zucchini
- 1 cup diced tomatoes
- Salt and pepper to taste
- Bread crumbs for topping (optional)

- Instructions:
    1. Cook macaroni according to package instructions. Drain and set aside.
    2. In a large pot, melt butter over medium heat. Whisk in flour until smooth.
    3. Gradually whisk in milk. Cook and stir until thickened and bubbly.
    4. Stir in shredded cheddar cheese until melted and smooth.
    5. Add cooked macaroni, diced bell peppers, diced zucchini, and diced tomatoes. Stir until well combined.
    6. Season with salt and pepper to taste.
    7. Optional: Sprinkle bread crumbs on top.
    8. Serve hot.

17. Sweet Potato and Black Bean Enchiladas
  - Ingredients:
    - 2 large sweet potatoes, peeled and diced
    - 1 can (15 oz) black beans, drained and rinsed
    - 1 onion, chopped
    - 2 garlic cloves, minced
    - 1 tbsp olive oil
    - 1 tbsp chili powder
    - 1 tsp cumin

- 1/2 tsp paprika
- Salt and pepper to taste
- 8 small flour tortillas
- 2 cups enchilada sauce
- 1 cup shredded cheddar cheese
- Fresh cilantro for garnish

- Instructions:
1. Preheat oven to 375°F (190°C). Grease a baking dish.
2. In a large skillet, heat olive oil over medium heat. Add chopped onion and minced garlic, cook until softened, about 5 minutes.
3. Add diced sweet potatoes, chili powder, cumin, paprika, salt, and pepper. Cook until sweet potatoes are tender, about 10 minutes.
4. Stir in black beans and cook for another 2-3 minutes.
5. Spoon the sweet potato and black bean mixture onto each tortilla. Roll up and place seam side down in the prepared baking dish.
6. Pour enchilada sauce over the rolled tortillas. Sprinkle with shredded cheddar cheese.
7. Bake for 20-25 minutes, or until cheese is melted and bubbly.
8. Serve hot, garnished with fresh cilantro.

18. Vegan Lentil Loaf
  - Ingredients:
    - 1 cup dry green or brown lentils
    - 3 cups vegetable broth
    - 1 onion, chopped
    - 2 garlic cloves, minced
    - 1 carrot, grated
    - 1 celery stalk, diced
    - 1/2 cup rolled oats
    - 1/4 cup ketchup
    - 2 tbsp soy sauce
    - 1 tsp dried thyme

- 1 tsp dried rosemary
- Salt and pepper to taste


- Instructions:
1. Preheat oven to 375°F (190°C). Grease a loaf pan.
2. In a saucepan, combine lentils and vegetable broth. Bring to a boil, then reduce heat and simmer for 20-25 minutes, until lentils are tender.
3. In a large skillet, heat olive oil over medium heat. Add chopped onion, minced garlic, grated carrot, and diced celery. Cook until vegetables are softened, about 5-7 minutes.
4. In a large bowl, combine cooked lentils, cooked vegetables, rolled oats, ketchup, soy sauce, dried thyme, dried rosemary, salt, and pepper. Mix until well combined.
5. Press the mixture into the prepared loaf pan.
6. Bake for 40-45 minutes, or until firm and golden brown on top.
7. Serve hot.


19. Butternut Squash and Sage Pasta
  - Ingredients:
    - 8 oz pasta of your choice
    - 2 cups butternut squash, diced
    - 2 tbsp olive oil
    - 2 garlic cloves, minced
    - 1/4 cup fresh sage leaves
    - 1/4 cup grated Parmesan cheese
    - Salt and pepper to taste


  - Instructions:
    1. Cook pasta according to package instructions. Drain and set aside.
    2. In a large skillet, heat olive oil over medium heat. Add diced butternut squash and cook until tender, about 10-15 minutes.

3. Add minced garlic and fresh sage leaves to the skillet. Cook for another 2-3 minutes, until fragrant.

4. Add cooked pasta to the skillet and toss to combine.

5. Stir in grated Parmesan cheese. Season with salt and pepper to taste.

6. Serve hot.


20. Baked Stuffed Acorn Squash
  - Ingredients:
    - 2 acorn squash, halved and seeds removed
    - 2 tbsp olive oil
    - 1 onion, chopped
    - 2 garlic cloves, minced
    - 1 cup cooked quinoa
    - 1 cup cooked black beans
    - 1/2 cup dried cranberries
    - 1/4 cup chopped pecans
    - 1 tsp dried sage
    - Salt and pepper to taste

  - Instructions:
    1. Preheat oven to 375°F (190°C). Place acorn squash

halves cut side down on a baking sheet. Bake for 30-40 minutes, or until tender.

2. In a large skillet, heat olive oil over medium heat. Add chopped onion and minced garlic, cook until softened, about 5 minutes.

3. Stir in cooked quinoa, cooked black beans, dried cranberries, chopped pecans, dried sage, salt, and pepper. Cook for another 2-3 minutes.

4. Spoon the quinoa mixture into the baked acorn squash halves.

5. Bake for another 10-15 minutes, or until heated through.

6. Serve hot.

# **Chapter 6: Sweet Treats**

1. Vegan Chocolate Avocado Mousse
   - Ingredients:
     - 2 ripe avocados
     - 1/2 cup cocoa powder
     - 1/2 cup maple syrup
     - 1/2 tsp vanilla extract
     - Pinch of salt
     - Fresh berries for garnish

   - Instructions:
     1. Scoop the flesh of the avocados into a blender or food processor.
     2. Add cocoa powder, maple syrup, vanilla extract, and a pinch of salt.
     3. Blend until smooth and creamy, scraping down the sides as needed.
     4. Spoon the mousse into serving dishes and refrigerate for at least 30 minutes.
     5. Serve chilled, garnished with fresh berries.

2. Baked Apples with Cinnamon and Walnuts
   - Ingredients:
     - 4 apples, cored
     - 1/4 cup chopped walnuts
     - 2 tbsp maple syrup
     - 1 tsp cinnamon
     - 1/4 cup water
     - Vanilla ice cream or yogurt for serving

   - Instructions:
     1. Preheat oven to 375°F (190°C).

2. In a bowl, combine chopped walnuts, maple syrup, and cinnamon.

3. Stuff each cored apple with the walnut mixture.

4. Place stuffed apples in a baking dish and pour water into the bottom of the dish.

5. Bake for 30-40 minutes, or until apples are tender.

6. Serve warm with a scoop of vanilla ice cream or yogurt.

3. Banana Oatmeal Cookies
  - Ingredients:
    - 2 ripe bananas, mashed
    - 1 cup rolled oats
    - 1/4 cup chopped nuts or chocolate chips
    - 1/4 tsp cinnamon
    - 1/4 tsp vanilla extract

  - Instructions:
      1. Preheat oven to 350°F (175°C). Line a baking sheet with parchment paper.

2. In a bowl, combine mashed bananas, rolled oats, chopped nuts or chocolate chips, cinnamon, and vanilla extract.

3. Drop spoonfuls of the mixture onto the prepared baking sheet.

4. Bake for 15-20 minutes, or until cookies are golden brown.

5. Allow to cool before serving.

4. Coconut Date Balls
  - Ingredients:
    - 1 cup dates, pitted
    - 1 cup shredded coconut
    - 1/4 cup almond butter
    - 1/4 cup chopped nuts (optional)
    - 1/4 tsp vanilla extract

- Instructions:
   1. Place dates in a food processor and process until they form a paste.
   2. Add shredded coconut, almond butter, chopped nuts, and vanilla extract. Process until well combined.
   3. Roll the mixture into small balls.
   4. Roll the balls in additional shredded coconut, if desired.
   5. Refrigerate for at least 30 minutes before serving.

5. Chia Seed Pudding
  - Ingredients:
    - 1/4 cup chia seeds
    - 1 cup almond milk
    - 1 tbsp maple syrup
    - 1/2 tsp vanilla extract
    - Fresh berries for topping

  - Instructions:
   1. In a bowl, combine chia seeds, almond milk, maple syrup, and vanilla extract.
   2. Stir well, then cover and refrigerate for at least 2 hours, or overnight.
   3. Stir the pudding before serving and top with fresh berries.

6. Baked Pears with Honey and Cinnamon
  - Ingredients:
    - 4 pears, halved and cored
    - 2 tbsp honey
    - 1 tsp cinnamon
    - 1/4 cup chopped nuts (e.g., walnuts, almonds)

  - Instructions:

1. Preheat oven to 375°F (190°C). Place pear halves cut side up in a baking dish.

2. Drizzle honey over the pears and sprinkle with cinnamon.

3. Bake for 30-40 minutes, or until pears are tender.

4. Sprinkle chopped nuts over the baked pears before serving.

7. Coconut Bliss Balls
   - Ingredients:
     - 1 cup shredded coconut
     - 1/2 cup almond flour
     - 1/4 cup maple syrup
     - 2 tbsp coconut oil, melted
     - 1 tsp vanilla extract
     - Pinch of salt

   - Instructions:
     1. In a bowl, mix shredded coconut, almond flour, maple syrup, melted coconut oil, vanilla extract, and a pinch of salt.

     2. Roll the mixture into balls and place on a baking sheet lined with parchment paper.

     3. Refrigerate for at least 30 minutes before serving.

8. Berry Parfait
   - Ingredients:
     - 1 cup Greek yogurt (or dairy-free alternative)
     - 1 cup mixed berries (e.g., strawberries, blueberries, raspberries)
     - 1/4 cup granola
     - 1 tbsp honey

   - Instructions:
     1. In a glass, layer Greek yogurt, mixed berries, and granola.
     2. Drizzle honey over the top before serving.

9. Chocolate-Dipped Strawberries
  - Ingredients:
    - 1 cup strawberries, washed and dried
    - 1/2 cup dark chocolate chips
    - 1 tsp coconut oil

  - Instructions:
    1. In a microwave-safe bowl, melt chocolate chips with coconut oil in 30-second intervals, stirring in between, until smooth.
    2. Dip each strawberry into the melted chocolate, covering about half of the strawberry.
    3. Place on a baking sheet lined with parchment paper and refrigerate until chocolate is set.

10. Apple Crisp
  - Ingredients:
    - 4 apples, peeled, cored, and sliced
    - 1 tbsp lemon juice
    - 1/2 cup rolled oats
    - 1/4 cup almond flour
    - 1/4 cup chopped nuts (e.g., pecans, walnuts)
    - 1/4 cup maple syrup
    - 2 tbsp coconut oil, melted
    - 1 tsp cinnamon
    - Pinch of salt

  - Instructions:
    1. Preheat oven to 350°F (175°C). Grease a baking dish.
    2. In a bowl, toss apple slices with lemon juice and spread them evenly in the baking dish.
    3. In a separate bowl, mix rolled oats, almond flour, chopped nuts, maple syrup, melted coconut oil, cinnamon, and a pinch of salt.
    4. Spread the oat mixture over the apples in the baking dish.

5. Bake for 30-40 minutes, or until apples are tender and topping is golden brown.

6. Serve warm.


11. Pumpkin Spice Muffins
  - Ingredients:
    - 1 3/4 cups all-purpose flour
    - 1 tsp baking soda
    - 1/2 tsp salt
    - 1 tsp cinnamon
    - 1/2 tsp nutmeg
    - 1/2 tsp cloves
    - 1/2 cup coconut oil, melted
    - 3/4 cup brown sugar
    - 1 can (15 oz) pumpkin puree
    - 2 eggs
    - 1 tsp vanilla extract
    - 1/2 cup chopped nuts (optional)

  - Instructions:
    1. Preheat oven to 375°F (190°C). Line a muffin tin with paper liners.

    2. In a bowl, whisk together flour, baking soda, salt, cinnamon, nutmeg, and cloves.

    3. In a separate bowl, mix melted coconut oil, brown sugar, pumpkin puree, eggs, and vanilla extract.

    4. Gradually add the dry ingredients to the wet ingredients, mixing until just combined.

    5. Fold in chopped nuts, if using.

    6. Fill each muffin cup with the batter.

    7. Bake for 20-25 minutes, or until a toothpick inserted into the center comes out clean.

    8. Allow to cool before serving.

12. Lemon Poppy Seed Loaf
   - Ingredients:
     - 1 1/2 cups all-purpose flour
     - 2 tbsp poppy seeds
     - 1 tsp baking powder
     - 1/2 tsp baking soda
     - 1/2 tsp salt
     - 1/2 cup unsalted butter, softened
     - 1 cup granulated sugar
     - 2 eggs
     - 1/2 cup Greek yogurt
     - Zest of 1 lemon
     - 2 tbsp lemon juice
     - 1 tsp vanilla extract

   - Instructions:
     1. Preheat oven to 350°F (175°C). Grease a loaf pan.
     2. In a bowl, whisk together flour, poppy seeds, baking powder, baking soda, and salt.
     3. In a separate bowl, cream together butter and sugar until light and fluffy.
     4. Beat in eggs, one at a time, then mix in Greek yogurt, lemon zest, lemon juice, and vanilla extract.
     5. Gradually add the dry ingredients to the wet ingredients, mixing until just combined.
     6. Pour the batter into the prepared loaf pan.
     7. Bake for 50-60 minutes, or until a toothpick inserted into the center comes out clean.
     8. Allow to cool before slicing.

13. Raspberry Chia Seed Jam
   - Ingredients:
     - 2 cups fresh or frozen raspberries

- 2 tbsp maple syrup
  - 2 tbsp chia seeds

- Instructions:
    1. In a saucepan, heat raspberries and maple syrup over medium heat, stirring occasionally, until raspberries break down and mixture begins to thicken.
    2. Stir in chia seeds and continue cooking for another 5 minutes.
    3. Remove from heat and let cool.
    4. Transfer to a jar and refrigerate for at least 1 hour before serving.

14. Chocolate Banana Bread
  - Ingredients:
    - 3 ripe bananas, mashed
    - 1/2 cup unsalted butter, melted
    - 1/2 cup Greek yogurt
    - 1/2 cup brown sugar
    - 1 egg
    - 1 tsp vanilla extract
    - 1 1/2 cups all-purpose flour
    - 1/4 cup cocoa powder
    - 1 tsp baking soda
    - 1/2 tsp salt
    - 1/2 cup chocolate chips

  - Instructions:
    1. Preheat oven to 350°F (175°C). Grease a loaf pan.
    2. In a bowl, mix mashed bananas, melted butter, Greek yogurt, brown sugar, egg, and vanilla extract.
    3. In a separate bowl, whisk together flour, cocoa powder, baking soda, and salt.
    4. Gradually add the dry ingredients to the wet ingredients, mixing until just combined.

5. Fold in chocolate chips.

6. Pour the batter into the prepared loaf pan.

7. Bake for 50-60 minutes, or until a toothpick inserted into the center comes out clean.

8. Allow to cool before slicing.

15. Coconut Macaroons
   - Ingredients:
     - 2 1/2 cups shredded coconut
     - 1/2 cup sweetened condensed milk
     - 1 tsp vanilla extract
     - 2 egg whites
     - Pinch of salt
     - Chocolate for dipping (optional)

   - Instructions:
     1. Preheat oven to 325°F (160°C). Line a baking sheet with parchment paper.

2. In a bowl, mix shredded coconut, sweetened condensed milk, and vanilla extract.

3. In a separate bowl, beat egg whites with a pinch of salt until stiff peaks form.

4. Gently fold the egg whites into the coconut mixture.

5. Drop spoonfuls of the mixture onto the prepared baking sheet.

6. Bake for 20-25 minutes, or until golden brown.

7. Allow to cool before serving.

8. Optional: Dip the bottoms of the macaroons in melted chocolate and let set.

16. Banana Ice Cream
   - Ingredients:
     - 4 ripe bananas, sliced and frozen
     - 1/4 cup milk or dairy-free alternative

- 1 tsp vanilla extract
  - Toppings of your choice (e.g., chocolate chips, nuts, fruit)

- Instructions:
  1. In a blender or food processor, blend frozen banana slices, milk, and vanilla extract until smooth and creamy.
  2. Serve immediately, topped with your favorite toppings.


17. Cinnamon Sugar Baked Donuts
  - Ingredients:
    - 1 cup all-purpose flour
    - 1/2 cup granulated sugar
    - 1 tsp baking powder
    - 1/2 tsp cinnamon
    - 1/4 tsp nutmeg
    - 1/2 cup milk
    - 1 egg
    - 1 tsp vanilla extract
    - 2 tbsp unsalted butter, melted
    - For coating: 1/4 cup unsalted butter, melted; 1/2 cup granulated sugar; 1 tsp cinnamon

  - Instructions:
    1. Preheat oven to 350°F (175°C). Grease a donut pan.
    2. In a bowl, whisk together flour, sugar, baking powder, cinnamon, and nutmeg.
    3. In a separate bowl, mix milk, egg, vanilla extract, and melted butter.
    4. Gradually add the wet ingredients to the dry ingredients, mixing until just combined.
    5. Spoon the batter into the prepared donut pan, filling each cavity about 2/3 full.

6. Bake for 10-12 minutes, or until donuts spring back when lightly pressed.

7. Allow donuts to cool in the pan for a few minutes, then transfer to a wire rack.

8. In a shallow bowl, mix granulated sugar and cinnamon for coating.

9. While donuts are still warm, brush each donut with melted butter, then dip into the cinnamon sugar mixture until coated.

10. Serve warm or at room temperature.

18. Blueberry Oat Bars
  - Ingredients:
    - 2 cups rolled oats
    - 1 cup all-purpose flour
    - 1/2 cup brown sugar
    - 1/2 tsp baking powder
    - 1/4 tsp salt
    - 1/2 cup unsalted butter, melted
    - 2 cups fresh or frozen blueberries
    - 1/4 cup granulated sugar
    - 2 tbsp lemon juice
    - Zest of 1 lemon

  - Instructions:
    1. Preheat oven to 350°F (175°C). Grease a 9x9-inch baking dish.

2. In a large bowl, mix rolled oats, flour, brown sugar, baking powder, and salt.

3. Stir in melted butter until mixture is crumbly.

4. Press half of the oat mixture into the bottom of the prepared baking dish.

5. In a separate bowl, mix blueberries, granulated sugar, lemon juice, and lemon zest.

6. Spread blueberry mixture over the oat layer in the baking dish.

7. Sprinkle the remaining oat mixture evenly over the blueberries.
8. Bake for 35-40 minutes, or until topping is golden brown.
9. Allow to cool before cutting into bars.

19. Peanut Butter Banana Bites
  - Ingredients:
    - 2 ripe bananas
    - 1/4 cup peanut butter
    - 1/4 cup chocolate chips
    - 1/4 cup chopped nuts (e.g., peanuts, almonds)
    - 1/4 cup shredded coconut (optional)

  - Instructions:
    1. Peel bananas and cut into bite-sized pieces.
    2. Spread peanut butter onto half of the banana pieces.
    3. Sandwich with the remaining banana pieces.
    4. Melt chocolate chips in the microwave in 30-second intervals, stirring in between, until smooth.
    5. Dip each banana bite halfway into the melted chocolate, then sprinkle with chopped nuts or shredded coconut, if desired.
    6. Place on a baking sheet lined with parchment paper and freeze until chocolate is set.
    7. Serve chilled.

20. Chocolate Zucchini Bread
  - Ingredients:
    - 1 1/2 cups all-purpose flour
    - 1/2 cup cocoa powder
    - 1 tsp baking soda
    - 1/2 tsp baking powder
    - 1/2 tsp salt
    - 1/2 cup unsalted butter, melted
    - 1/2 cup granulated sugar

- 1/2 cup brown sugar
- 2 eggs
- 1 tsp vanilla extract
- 1 1/2 cups grated zucchini
- 1/2 cup chocolate chips

- Instructions:
1. Preheat oven to 350°F (175°C). Grease a loaf pan.
2. In a bowl, whisk together flour, cocoa powder, baking soda, baking powder, and salt.
3. In a separate bowl, mix melted butter, granulated sugar, brown sugar, eggs, and vanilla extract until smooth.
4. Gradually add the dry ingredients to the wet ingredients, mixing until just combined.
5. Fold in grated zucchini and chocolate chips.
6. Pour the batter into the prepared loaf pan.
7. Bake for 50-60 minutes, or until a toothpick inserted into the center comes out clean.
8. Allow to cool before slicing.

# Chapter 7: 4 weeks meal plan

Week 1

- Day 1
  - Breakfast: Vegan Chocolate Avocado Mousse
  - Lunch: Quinoa-Stuffed Acorn Squash
  - Dinner: Sweet Potato and Black Bean Tacos
- Day 2
  - Breakfast: Berry Chia Seed Pudding
  - Lunch: Lentil and Vegetable Soup
  - Dinner: Baked Salmon with Lemon and Dill
- Day 3
  - Breakfast: Blueberry Oat Bars
  - Lunch: Mediterranean Chickpea Salad
  - Dinner: Coconut Curry Lentils
- Day 4
  - Breakfast: Pumpkin Spice Muffins
  - Lunch: Spinach and Strawberry Salad
  - Dinner: Vegetable Stir-Fry with Tofu
- Day 5
  - Breakfast: Banana-Oat Cookies
  - Lunch: Roasted Vegetable Wrap
  - Dinner: Lentil Bolognese with Zucchini Noodles
- Day 6
  - Breakfast: Apple Cinnamon Overnight Oats
  - Lunch: Greek Quinoa Salad
  - Dinner: Stuffed Bell Peppers with Quinoa and Black Beans
- Day 7
  - Breakfast: Chocolate Banana Bread
  - Lunch: Avocado and White Bean Wrap
  - Dinner: Lentil and Sweet Potato Shepherd's Pie

Week 2

- Day 1
  - Breakfast: Lemon Poppy Seed Loaf
  - Lunch: Quinoa Salad with Roasted Vegetables
  - Dinner: Baked Chicken with Herbs
- Day 2
  - Breakfast: Peanut Butter Banana Bites
  - Lunch: Lentil and Kale Salad
  - Dinner: Mushroom Risotto
- Day 3
  - Breakfast: Coconut Bliss Balls
  - Lunch: Caprese Sandwich with Pesto
  - Dinner: Cauliflower and Chickpea Curry
- Day 4
  - Breakfast: Chocolate Zucchini Bread
  - Lunch: Greek Lentil Soup
  - Dinner: Spaghetti Squash with Marinara Sauce
- Day 5
  - Breakfast: Almond Butter Energy Balls
  - Lunch: Quinoa and Black Bean Stuffed Peppers
  - Dinner: Sweet Potato and Lentil Curry
- Day 6
  - Breakfast: Baked Apple Oatmeal
  - Lunch: Mediterranean Quinoa Bowl
  - Dinner: Baked Cod with Tomato and Basil
- Day 7
  - Breakfast: Banana Ice Cream
  - Lunch: Roasted Vegetable and Hummus Wrap
  - Dinner: Chickpea and Vegetable Tagine

Week 3

- Day 1
  - Breakfast: Vegan Chocolate Avocado Mousse
  - Lunch: Lentil and Vegetable Soup
  - Dinner: Stuffed Bell Peppers with Quinoa and Black Beans
- Day 2
  - Breakfast: Berry Chia Seed Pudding
  - Lunch: Mediterranean Chickpea Salad
  - Dinner: Lentil Bolognese with Zucchini Noodles
- Day 3
  - Breakfast: Blueberry Oat Bars
  - Lunch: Spinach and Strawberry Salad
  - Dinner: Coconut Curry Lentils
- Day 4
  - Breakfast: Pumpkin Spice Muffins
  - Lunch: Lentil and Kale Salad
  - Dinner: Mushroom Risotto
- Day 5
  - Breakfast: Banana-Oat Cookies
  - Lunch: Quinoa Salad with Roasted Vegetables
  - Dinner: Baked Salmon with Lemon and Dill
- Day 6
  - Breakfast: Apple Cinnamon Overnight Oats
  - Lunch: Greek Quinoa Salad
  - Dinner: Cauliflower and Chickpea Curry
- Day 7
  - Breakfast: Chocolate Banana Bread
  - Lunch: Caprese Sandwich with Pesto
  - Dinner: Sweet Potato and Lentil Curry

Week 4

- Day 1
  - Breakfast: Lemon Poppy Seed Loaf
  - Lunch: Roasted Vegetable Wrap
  - Dinner: Lentil and Sweet Potato Shepherd's Pie
- Day 2
  - Breakfast: Peanut Butter Banana Bites
  - Lunch: Lentil and Vegetable Soup
  - Dinner: Chickpea and Vegetable Tagine
- Day 3
  - Breakfast: Coconut Bliss Balls
  - Lunch: Greek Lentil Soup
  - Dinner: Stuffed Bell Peppers with Quinoa and Black Beans
- Day 4
  - Breakfast: Chocolate Zucchini Bread
  - Lunch: Mediterranean Quinoa Bowl
  - Dinner: Sweet Potato and Black Bean Tacos
- Day 5
  - Breakfast: Almond Butter Energy Balls
  - Lunch: Quinoa-Stuffed Acorn Squash
  - Dinner: Baked Cod with Tomato and Basil
- Day 6
  - Breakfast: Baked Apple Oatmeal
  - Lunch: Spinach and Strawberry Salad
  - Dinner: Mushroom Risotto
- Day 7
  - Breakfast: Banana Ice Cream
  - Lunch: Lentil and Kale Salad
  - Dinner: Coconut Curry Lentils

# Conclusion:

In conclusion, this cookbook, "Rheumatoid Arthritis Cookbook for Women: Wholesome Recipes to Manage Inflammatory Flare-ups and Fatigue," has been crafted with care to provide nourishing and delicious meals that support women living with rheumatoid arthritis. The recipes included in this cookbook are designed to not only delight your taste buds but also to help you manage the symptoms of rheumatoid arthritis through the power of nutritious food.

By focusing on ingredients that are known to have anti-inflammatory properties and avoiding those that may exacerbate inflammation, these recipes aim to provide relief and support for women dealing with the challenges of rheumatoid arthritis. Whether you're looking for hearty and comforting meals or light and refreshing snacks, this cookbook has something for every craving and occasion.

We hope that the recipes in this cookbook will inspire you to explore new flavors and cooking techniques while also providing you with the tools you need to take control of your health and well-being. Remember, managing rheumatoid arthritis is about more than just what you eat – it's about nourishing your body and soul to thrive despite the challenges you may face.

Thank you for allowing us to be a part of your journey toward better health. Here's to a future filled with good food, good health, and good living.